21904

D1388143

The Library, Education Centre
Royal Surrey County Hospital
Egerton Road, Guildford, GU2 7XX
Tel: 01483 464137

Class number   WG 540

Computer number   H0606140.

VENOUS THROMBOSIS IN WOMEN

*Pregnancy, The Contraceptive Pill and
Hormone Replacement Therapy*

VENOUS THROMBOSIS IN WOMEN

Pregnancy, The Contraceptive Pill and Hormone Replacement Therapy

I. A. Greer

Regius Professor of Obstetrics and Gynaecology
Head, Division of Developmental Medicine
University of Glasgow
Glasgow Royal Infirmary, Glasgow, UK

The Parthenon Publishing Group
International Publishers in Medicine, Science & Technology

A CRC PRESS COMPANY
BOCA RATON   LONDON   NEW YORK   WASHINGTON, D.C.

Published in the USA by
The Parthenon Publishing Group
345 Park Avenue South, 10th Floor
New York, NY 10010
USA

Published in the UK and Europe by
The Parthenon Publishing Group
23–25 Blades Court
Deodar Road
London SW15 2NU
UK

Copyright © 2003 The Parthenon Publishing Group

Library of Congress Cataloging-in-Publication Data
Data available on request

British Library Cataloguing in Publication Data
Greer, I. A. (Ian A.)
    Venous thrombosis in women: pregnancy, the contraceptive pill and hormone
    replacement therapy
    1. Thrombophlebitis 2. Women - Diseases
    I. Title
    616.1'45'0082

ISBN 1-84214-228-3

First published in 2003

*No part of this book may be reproduced in any form without permission from the
publishers except for the quotation of brief passages for the purposes of review*

Composition by The Parthenon Publishing Group
Printed and bound in the USA

Contents

1

Overview of the hemostatic and fibrinolytic systems

Physiologically, the hemostatic and fibrinolytic systems maintain vascular integrity, ensuring the circulation of blood within the vascular tree. In the pathological situation, they will repair damage to the vessel wall, sealing the defect induced by injury or disease. Failure of the regulatory systems balancing the hemostatic and fibrinolytic systems can lead to thrombosis or excessive bleeding. The endothelium is a key factor in the regulation of hemostasis and fibrinolysis, and also vasomotor tone. These dynamic processes are augmented by the structural barrier provided by the endothelium, separating blood from the tissue elements which will activate coagulation, in the vessel wall.

Following vascular injury, vasoconstriction, mediated through potent endothelial and platelet-derived vasoconstrictors such as endothelin and thromboxane A_2, respectively, minimizes blood loss. At the same time, primary hemostasis occurs. This is the formation of a platelet plug. Platelets are activated by tissue components in the subendothelial structure such as collagen, as well as the release of platelet adhesive molecules on the endothelial surface including von Willebrand's factor. Platelet activation also plays a key role in facilitating activation of the coagulation system by exposing receptors on the platelet surface for specific clotting factors, particularly factor Va which, along with anionic surface phospholipids on the cell membrane, following activation provides a catalytic surface facilitating the conversion of prothrombin to thrombin by factor Xa. Platelet activation is also effected by thrombin generated in the secondary hemostatic response[1,2].

The secondary hemostatic response to injury is the formation of fibrin around the platelet plug, helping to attach it firmly to the vessel wall. The secondary response is triggered by the expression of tissue factor on the endothelial surface at the site of injury. Tissue factor (TF), also known as thromboplastin, acts as a cofactor for the plasma serine protease, activated factor VII (FVIIa), and is the most potent initiator known of the coagulation pathway. Ninety-nine per cent of FVII circulates as the zymogen or unactivated form, and around 1% circulates as FVIIa, the activated form. Both FVII and FVIIa are bound to TF expressed on the vessel wall, thus localizing the hemostatic response. Once FVII binds to TF, it can be activated by TF itself, thrombin, activated factor IX (FIXa) and activated factor X (FXa). The FVIIa–TF complex triggers further activation of the coagulation system by two mechanisms. First, it will activate factor X directly, and, second, it will activate FIX which, in concert with its protein cofactor activated factor VIII, will convert factor X to its active form FXa. All these reactions occur on phospholipid surfaces such as those provided by activated platelets. The factor Xa, again on a phospholipid surface, then assembles with its cofactor factor Va, to generate thrombin from prothrombin (factor II). The final step in the pathway is the conversion of fibrinogen to fibrin by thrombin, with release of fibrinopeptides. Initially, the fibrinogen, a large glycoprotein with a molecular weight of 340 000 present in plasma and also released from activated platelets, undergoes hydrolysis and forms fibrin monomers. These fibrin monomers in turn undergo spontaneous polymerization, to provide a fibrin clot at the site of vascular injury. Following the initial generation of the fibrin clot, covalent cross-linking of the fibrin monomers by activated factor XIII occurs (factor XIII is itself activated by thrombin), and this reduces its susceptibility to breakdown by the fibrinolytic system (Figure 1.1)[3,4].

Clearly, thrombin plays a pivotal role in the regulation of hemostasis and fibrinolysis. Not only does it generate fibrin from fibrinogen and activate platelets, it can also amplify the hemostatic response by activating factors V and VIII, trigger fibrinolysis by stimulating release of tissue plasminogen activator from the endothelium, and activate one of the endogenous anticoagulant pathways by binding to thrombomodulin on the endothelial cell, leading to activation of protein C, an inhibitor of coagulation.

This hemostatic system is counterbalanced by the endogenous antithrombotic and fibrinolytic systems. These systems, along with hemodilution and blood flow, localize the hemostatic response. Antithrombotic factors expressed by the vessel wall are important in preventing platelet and neutrophil activation, and cell adhesion to the endothelial surface. Expression of anticoagulant glycosaminoglycans, such as heparan sulfate, on the cell surface and secretion of prostacyclin

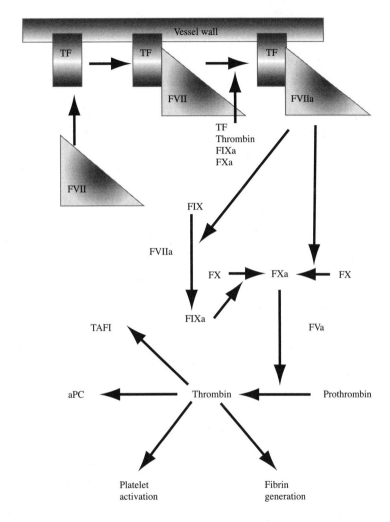

Figure 1.1   The hemostatic system. The key step in activation of the hemostatic system is the interaction of factor VII (FVII) and tissue factor (TF). Ninety-nine percent of FVII circulates in the zymogen or unactivated form and around 1% circulates as FVIIa, the activated form. When TF is expressed on the vessel wall owing to injury, it binds with FVII and FVIIa. Once FVII binds to TF, it can be activated by TF itself, thrombin, activated factor IX (FIXa) and activated factor X (FXa). The TF–FVIIa complex activates FX directly and also indirectly through activation of FIX acting with activated factor VIII (FVIIIa). FXa, acting with activated factor V (FVa), then converts prothrombin (factor II) to thrombin (factor IIa). Thrombin will convert fibrinogen to fibrin, and will also activate platelets, enhancing the reaction. Thrombin also stimulates activation of the protein C (aPC) anticoagulant system and thrombin-activated fibrinolytic inhibitor (TAFI)

and nitric oxide help to maintain the vessel's thromboresistant properties.

There are two endogenous circulating anticoagulant systems: the antithrombin and protein C/protein S systems. Antithrombin is a member of the serpin (serine proteinase inhibitor) gene family. The name antithrombin is something of a misnomer as it inactivates many serine proteases, not just thrombin, in the coagulation cascade, including factors Xa, IXa, XIa, XIIa and FVIIa–TF. There are two key reactive sites on the antithrombin molecule: the reactive site at the amino terminus of the molecule and the heparin binding site. Thrombin cleaves the reactive site followed by the formation of a thrombin–antithrombin complex that is rapidly cleared from the circulation. Heparin alters the structure of the antithrombin molecule, markedly enhancing its ability to bind these activated coagulation factors. As well as acting on the developing thrombus, antithrombin acts as a circulating scavenger for thrombin, and it may play a crucial role in regulating low levels of coagulation activation such as occurs in pregnancy. Thrombin–antithrombin (TAT) complexes are cleared by the liver through specific binding primarily to low-density lipoprotein receptor related protein (LRP).

The protein C/protein S system, which is largely regulated through thrombin generation as noted above, provides negative feedback to the coagulation cascade and so prevents excessive procoagulant activity. Protein C and protein S are vitamin K-dependent proteins produced by the liver. Protein C circulates as a zymogen. Although it can be activated directly by thrombin, activation is more efficient when thrombin binds to thrombomodulin on the vessel wall. Following activation by the thrombin–thrombomodulin complex, protein C, along with its cofactor protein S, inactivates factors Va and VIIIa through proteolytic cleavage. The factor Va inactivation occurs via an ordered series of 'cuts' in the factor V molecule's heavy chain; initially, there is a rapid 'cut' at Arg506, then slower rates of cleavage at two more sites (Arg306 and Arg679). Protein S enhances by around 20-fold the rate of the slower cleavage steps, and also enhances the affinity of protein C to bind to negatively charged phospholipids.

The fibrinolytic system balances the hemostatic system through its ability to break down fibrin. Breakdown of fibrin is effected through the actions of plasmin, a trypsin-like proteinase, which is derived from the α-globulin plasminogen, a plasma zymogen with a molecular weight of 90 kDa[5]. The conversion of plasminogen to plasmin is regulated by plasminogen activators, which are released from activated endothelial cells. There are two activators: tissue plasminogen activator (t-PA) and urokinase-type plasminogen activator (u-PA) (Figure 1.2). Constitutional deficiency of plasmin and its activators can lead to thrombotic problems. Plasmin will also help to amplify the fibrinolytic response by cleavage of an activation peptide from plasminogen, converting Glu-plasminogen to Lys-plasminogen. Lys-plasminogen has a greater affinity for fibrin than the parent molecule Glu-plasminogen, and is more susceptible to activation by plasminogen activators. During fibrin formation, t-PA and plasminogen, released by endothelial cells in response to thrombin, bind to fibrin. Indeed, plasminogen is more reactive when bound to fibrin by its lysine binding sites. Thus, both the activation factor and the plasminogen zymogen are present in the fibrin clot. This facilitates fibrinolysis when the system is fully activated. However, platelets and endothelial cells also release plasminogen activator inhibitor type 1 (PAI-1), and α_2-plasmin inhibitor when activated. Both PAI-1 and α_2-plasmin inhibitor bind to fibrin, and so fibrinolysis is impaired in the early stages of fibrin clot formation. This allows the integrity of the fibrin clot to be maintained in the early stages of the hemostatic response[4].

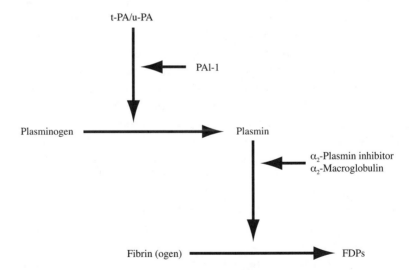

Figure 1.2 The fibrinolytic pathway. t-PA, tissue plasminogen activator; u-PA, urokinase-type plasminogen activator; PAI-1, plasminogen activator inhibitor type 1; FDPs, fibrinogen degradation products

Circulating plasmin does not usually have any effect on circulating fibrinogen owing to the presence of α_2-plasmin inhibitor in the circulation. This single-chain glycoprotein, which is the most important inhibitor of plasmin, rapidly forms a 1 : 1 complex with plasmin by binding to the lysine binding sites on the plasmin. This immediately neutralizes the activity of any plasmin in the circulation, as the lysine binding sites are also where fibrin is non-covalently bound to plasmin. In addition, plasmin cleaves the reactive site of α_2-plasmin inhibitor, resulting in a covalent plasmin–α_2-plasmin inhibitor complex. Thus, α_2-plasmin inhibitor helps to limit the plasmin-mediated fibrinolytic response to a local thrombus by competitively inhibiting the binding of plasminogen to fibrin. Interestingly, constitutional deficiency of α_2-plasmin inhibitor will result in the hemostatic fibrin plug being dissolved before healing has occurred, with resultant hemorrhagic problems. A second plasma protein, α_2-macroglubin, can also inhibit plasmin, but this acts more as a 'back-up' system for α_2-plasmin inhibitor (Figure 1.2)[5].

Plasminogen activators are inhibited by PAI-1. This is released by endothelial cells and platelets following their activation. It complexes with and neutralizes t-PA[6]. Constitutional deficiency of PAI-1 can result in bleeding problems. There is also a second type of plasminogen activator inhibitor that is produced and released from the placenta (PAI-2). This is an important inhibitor of fibrinolysis in pregnancy, where there is physiological down-regulation of the fibrinolytic system. α_2-Plasmin inhibitor also inhibits plasminogen activators; specifically, fibrin-bound α_2-plasmin inhibitor can inhibit fibrin-bound t-PA, providing local inhibition of fibrinolysis[7]. In addition, thrombin generated by the hemostatic system will activate a proenzyme, thrombin-activated fibrinolytic inhibitor (TAFI), so providing a further regulatory system that can impair the fibrinolytic attack on fibrin (Figure 1.1). TAFI cleaves plasminogen-binding sites (C-terminal lysine residues) from fibrinogen, thus promoting stabilization of fibrin and providing a more persistent clot. TAFI also inhibits the conversion of Glu-plasminogen to Lys-plasminogen. Thus, in the early stages of hemostatic system activation, the overall balance between the hemostatic and fibrinolytic systems will be in favor of fibrin generation, particularly, through the effects of TAFI. Gradually, the balance switches in favor of fibrinolysis, and the fibrin strands are broken down into fibrin degradation products (FDPs) (Figure 1.2). These FDPs in turn can inhibit thrombin's action

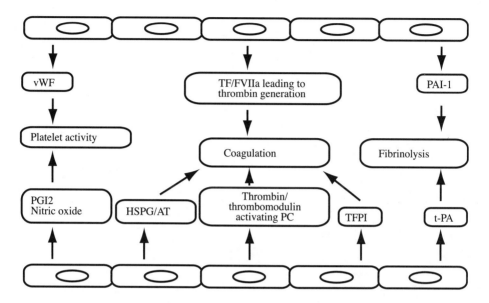

Figure 1.3   Schematic representation summarizing some of the prothrombotic and antithrombotic mechanisms regulated by the vascular endothelium. The upper part illustrates the prothrombic effects of the endothelium: release of von Willebrand factor (vWF) to activate platelets; stimulation of coagulation through tissue factor expression and activation of FVII leading, through the coagulation cascade, to thrombin generation, and inhibition of fibrinolysis through PAI-1. The lower part shows the antithrombotic effects of the endothelium; release of heparin-like substances (heparan sulfate proteoglycan [HSPG]) that enhance the activity of antithrombin (AT); thrombomodulin expression which binds thrombin and enhances activation of protein C (PC); release of tissue factor pathway inhibitor (TFPI); and release of tissue plasminogen activator which inhibits fibrinolysis

and also inhibit fibrin polymerization, and therefore have an anticoagulant effect, a phenomenon perhaps best known in disseminated intravascular coagulation. The complex interactions between the coagulation and fibrinolytic pathways mean that dysfunction of one pathway interacts with the other. This is particularly true in relation to thrombin, which orchestrates many aspects of hemostasis and fibrinolysis. For example, in hemophilia with factor VIII deficiency, not only are thrombin generation and coagulation impaired, but also there is reduced TAFI release making any clot that does form more susceptible to breakdown, so enhancing the bleeding problem. The converse applies for patients with thrombophilia, where excess thrombin and TAFI production may allow a more fibrinolytic resistant clot to form (Figure 1.3).

2
Physiological changes in hemostasis and fibrinolysis in pregnancy

2.1 PLATELETS IN PREGNANCY

The weight of evidence favors a modest reduction in platelet count in pregnancy towards term[8–12]. Burrows and Kelton[11] studied over 1300 subjects and found a mean platelet count at term of 225 x 10⁹/l (95% confidence interval 109–341 × 10⁹/l), which is below accepted non-pregnant normal values. The reports of increased mean platelet volume and volume distribution width[13,14] are consistent with a compensated state of progressive platelet destruction, particularly during the third trimester. However, a cytofluorimetry study[15], using an antibody directed against a platelet α granule membrane protein to identify activated platelets *ex vivo*, observed no platelet volume change or activation. *In vitro*, an increase in platelet reactivity is seen in normal pregnancy in response to a variety of agonists that stimulate aggregation, but particularly those that are thromboxane-dependent[16–20]. This may reflect increased platelet sensitivity to thromboxane A2[21], and a relative failure of increased cyclic adenosine monophosphate (cAMP) production in response to agents such as prostacyclin, which inhibit platelet function through cAMP[21]. An increase in circulating platelet aggregates also suggests a degree of *in vivo* platelet activation in normal pregnancy[22], in keeping with enhanced reactivity, while *ex vivo* platelet reactivity is simultaneously reduced. This apparent paradox may reflect a degree of platelet exhaustion consequent upon enhanced activation *in vivo*. *In vivo* platelet activation is also supported by increased plasma levels of β-thromboglobulin, a protein reflecting *in vivo* platelet activation and degranulation[23]. Thus, the available evidence is consistent with a degree of enhanced platelet activation and/or destruction in normal pregnancy, which is partly compensated by increased production, thus resulting in a reduction in platelet count. Following delivery, the platelet count increases[9] in reaction to, and in compensation for, platelet consumption.

2.2 COAGULATION FACTORS

Factor XIIc increases in pregnancy, factor XIc remains essentially static and factor IXc may increase slightly[24]. Factor Xc, factor VIIIc and von Willebrand factor antigen increase progressively as pregnancy advances[8,24], with a parallel increase in ristocetin cofactor activity, the functional assessment of von Willebrand factor[24]. Factor VII and factor Vc also increase[8], while prothrombin does not change[8,24]. Fibrinogen increases substantially and progressively with gestation; a significant change is evident from the first trimester, and an almost two-fold increase over non-pregnant levels by term[8,9,24]. Factor XIII shows an initial increase but then falls to normal non-pregnant values in late pregnancy[25]. Overall, there is a marked increase in the coagulation potential, which is maximal around term. As this is associated with an increase in prothrombin fragments F1 + 2, and thrombin–antithrombin complexes indicating thrombin generation from prothrombin by the action of factor Xa *in vivo*[12,24,26], this increase in potential is, in part, accompanied by increased activation of the coagulation system and thrombin generation *in vivo* during pregnancy. Indeed, the increases in prothrombin fragments F1 + 2, and thrombin–antithrombin complexes are not dissimilar to those seen after a thromboembolic event[27], emphasizing the known association of pregnancy and venous thrombosis. Interestingly, however, a recent study assessing the expression of tissue factor (TF) on monocytes has shown that there is down-regulation of TF expression during pregnancy (TF is expressed not only on the endothelium but also on monocytes, in particular in response to stimuli such as proinflammatory cytokines). It has been proposed that this down-regulation may represent a compensatory mechanism for the previously described procoagulant changes in the hemostatic system during pregnancy[28].

2.3 ENDOGENOUS ANTICOAGULANTS AND PREGNANCY

The endogenous inhibitor of coagulation, antithrombin, is not altered by pregnancy[8,24]. Protein C levels remain constant[24]. Protein S exists in plasma in two forms: the functionally active free protein S and protein S complexed with C4b-binding protein, which is functionally inactive as it cannot interact with activated protein C. Normally, an equilibrium exists in plasma between these two forms. In normal pregnancy, there is a significant reduction in protein S activity[24], and this appears to be due to a reduction in total protein S as measured antigenically rather than a change in C4b-binding protein[29] (Figure 2.1).

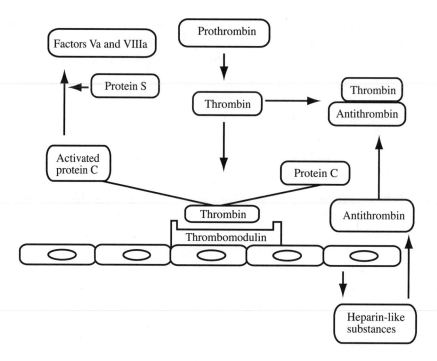

Figure 2.1   Schematic representation of the endogenous anticoagulant systems. Thrombin, generated from prothrombin by the coagulation cascade, is inactivated by binding to antithrombin. The activity of antithrombin against thrombin is markedly enhanced by heparin, and heparin-like substances released from the endothelium. Thrombin also binds to a receptor, thrombomodulin, on the endothelial surface. This complex enhances the activation of protein C by thrombin. The activated protein C, along with its cofactor protein S, breaks down activated factor V (FVa) and activated factor VIIIa (FVIIIa) by proteolytic cleavage

2.4 FIBRINOLYSIS

Overall, fibrinolytic activity is impaired during pregnancy, but returns rapidly to normal following delivery[8,26,30]. This is due largely to placentally derived plasminogen activator inhibitor type 2 (PAI-2), which is present in substantial quantities during pregnancy[31–33]. The endothelial derived inhibitor of plasminogen activator (PAI-1) also increases in pregnancy, by around three-fold[26]. These changes in PAI-1 and PAI-2 may be important for local deposition of fibrin in the placental bed, which is important for the physiological adaptation of pregnancy.

Plasminogen increases during pregnancy[9,34,35] as does antiplasmin, and tissue plasminogen activator, which is derived from the endothelium, increases by around two-fold[26]. Despite the reduction in fibrinolytic activity, fibrinolysis cannot be completely shut down as fibrin degradation products remain in the plasma and indeed increase as pregnancy advances[8]. D-dimer, a specific marker of fibrinolysis resulting from the breakdown of cross-linked fibrin polymer by plasmin, increases as pregnancy progresses[12]. Thrombin-activated fibrinolytic inhibitor (TAFI) levels also increase moderately throughout pregnancy, but, although TAFI levels increase, they do not show an inverse correlation with D-dimer levels[36]. The activity of the fibrinolytic system in response to stimulation of fibrinolysis by venous occlusion has been assessed in pregnancy. Total tissue plasminogen activator (t-PA) release is significantly reduced in pregnancy, with free t-PA remaining below the limit of detection of the assay following occlusion[37]. This is in contrast to the non-pregnant situation where both total and free t-PA increase significantly following venous occlusion. These data suggest that t-PA release is impaired in pregnancy and that free t-PA is rapidly inhibited, in keeping with the high levels of plasminogen activator inhibitors noted in pregnancy. Despite this impairment in the response to venous occlusion, D-dimer fragments of cross-linked fibrin are substantially increased in the first, second and third trimesters as compared with non-pregnant women[37]. This indicates that fibrinolysis is still occurring, and that it is not impaired to the extent suggested by the reduced levels of t-PA and increased levels of PAI-1 and PAI-2. However, the increase in D-dimer is likely to reflect an increase in fibrin production, as discussed above, rather than enhanced fibrinolysis. Impaired fibrinolysis can be found in some patients with a history of deep venous thrombosis[38], and the physiological impairment of fibrinolysis seen in pregnancy may contribute to the increased thrombotic risk associated with pregnancy.

2.5 SUMMARY: HEMOSTASIS IN NORMAL PREGNANCY

Overall, the data discussed in relation to changes in the coagulation and fibrinolytic systems in pregnancy indicate that there is a degree of activation of both systems, with generation of fibrin and subsequent fibrinolysis with increased levels of fibrinogen degradation products (FDPs) such as D-dimer. These changes are compatible with a compensated state of low-grade disseminated intravascular coagulation. This is supported by other studies where increased fibrinopeptide A, FDPs and platelet release products have been found in normal pregnancies indicating coagulation, fibrinolysis and *in vivo* platelet activation, respectively[39], in keeping with compensated low-grade disseminated intravascular coagulation. It is interesting that the above study found that fibrinectin levels were not increased, indicating that, despite the low-grade disseminated intravascular coagulation, there was no evidence of endothelial damage, in contrast to disorders such as pre-eclampsia where low grade disseminated intravascular coagulation is associated with endothelial injury.

The mechanism(s) underlying these physiological changes is (are) unclear. One possibility is that these changes are effected through the physiological changes in steroid hormones seen in pregnancy. It is clear that exogenous estrogen, such as in the oral contraceptive pill and hormone replacement therapy, can promote changes in coagulation and fibrinolysis[40–42], some of which are similar to those seen in pregnancy. Another possibility is the physiological hyperlipidemia of pregnancy[43], which can also promote changes in coagulation and fibrinolysis[44–46] such as increases in factor VIIa, fibrinogen and plasminogen activator inhibitor, albeit that the changes in lipid metabolism could themselves be brought about through estrogen. Such changes in lipid metabolism can also influence endothelial function, which plays a pivotal role in the control of coagulation and fibrinolysis[47].

3

Venous thromboembolism in pregnancy

3.1 THE PROBLEM OF VENOUS THROMBOEMBOLISM IN PREGNANCY

Pulmonary thromboembolism (PTE) remains a major cause of maternal mortality, and is currently the most common direct cause of maternal death in the United Kingdom[48]. Deep venous thrombosis (DVT) underlies PTE. Many DVTs leading to fatal PTE are not recognized clinically, being identified only at post-mortem examination following a maternal death. As well as the acute morbidity and mortality of venous thromboembolism (VTE) in pregnancy, DVT is associated with a significant risk of recurrent venous thrombosis and deep venous insufficiency, while PTE carries a risk of subsequent pulmonary hypertension. Pregnancy-related VTE may also identify women with an underlying thrombophilia, with implications not only for venous thrombosis but also for an increased risk of pregnancy complications such as pre-eclampsia and intrauterine growth restriction (IUGR).

The UK Confidential Enquiries into maternal deaths have shown that the overall incidence of fatal PTE has fallen substantially from the early 1950s (Figure 3.1). However, the greatest reduction has been in the number of deaths following vaginal delivery, which is probably

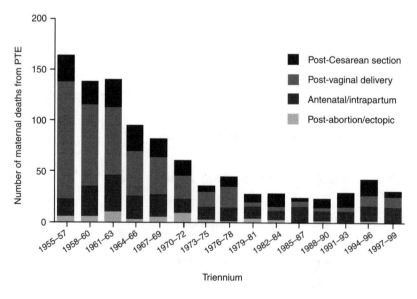

Figure 3.1   Incidence of fatal pulmonary thromboembolism (PTE) in England and Wales, 1955–84 and the UK, 1985–99

related to the 'de-medicalization' of childbirth, with shorter stays in hospital and more rapid mobilization as well as shorter labors. None the less, in recent years, there has been no further reduction in fatalities after vaginal delivery[48], and the number of deaths during the antenatal period has changed little from the early 1950s despite major advances in identification of risk, thromboprophylaxis, diagnosis and therapeutics over this same period. The total number of deaths following Cesarean section fell sharply in the most recent report; this may reflect the widespread introduction of specific thromboprophylaxis to UK clinical obstetric practice in the mid-1990s. The need for adequate diagnosis and treatment of thromboembolic disease in pregnancy has been highlighted by the UK Confidential Enquiries into Maternal Deaths[48]. It is clear that many of these deaths are associated with substandard care, including a failure to recognize risk factors for VTE, a failure to provide appropriate thromboprophylaxis for those at risk, a failure to diagnose VTE objectively and a failure to provide appropriate treatment. Specifically, the recent increase in fatalities after vaginal delivery[48] has highlighted the need for thromboprophylaxis following vaginal delivery in women at increased risk.

The incidence of clinically evident antenatal DVT has been estimated from a Scottish National study of a cohort of over 600 000 maternities to be 0.615/1000 maternities in women under 35 years of age, and 1.216/1000 maternities in women over 35 years of age[49]. In this same study, the incidence of postpartum DVT has been estimated at 0.304/1000 maternities in women under 35 years of age and 0.72/1000 maternities in women over 35 years of age (Figure 3.2). Although antenatal DVT is more common than postpartum DVT[49,50], the event rate is higher in the 6 weeks of the puerperium, making it the time of greatest risk. Almost 40% of postpartum DVTs present following the woman's discharge from hospital, but complete data on postpartum DVT are difficult to obtain as many cases present to nonobstetric services. The UK Confidential Enquiries, however, provide accurate data for fatal PTE.

3.2 RISK FACTORS FOR VTE IN PREGNANCY

In order to provide prophylaxis for thromboembolism, an assessment of the woman's risk must be made ideally pre-pregnancy or in early

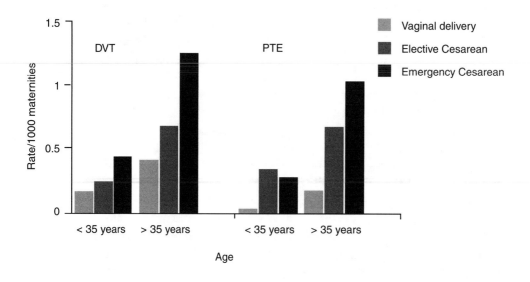

Figure 3.2   Incidence of deep vein thrombosis (DVT) and pulmonary thromboembolism (PTE) after vaginal delivery and elective and emergency Cesarean section and the interaction with age over 35 years[49]

pregnancy. Identification of increased risk is usually straightforward and easily assessed in the clinic. The common risk factors for VTE in pregnancy are: age over 35 years, obesity, operative delivery (especially emergency Cesarean section in labor), thrombophilia, and a family or personal history of thrombosis suggestive of an underlying thrombophilia[51]. Additional risk factors include gross varicose veins, immobility, paraplegia, dehydration, infective and inflammatory conditions such as inflammatory bowel disease and urinary tract infection, preeclampsia, major obstetric hemorrhage such as abruption, intravenous drug abuse, and concomitant medical conditions such as nephrotic syndrome where loss of antithrombin in the proteinuria may provoke an acquired deficiency in antithrombin and increased risk of VTE. A significant proportion of VTEs occur in the first trimester, and it should be noted that problems such as hyperemesis where the woman may be dehydrated and immobile represents a significant risk. Increasingly, long distance travel is seen as an important risk factor (Table 3.1).

Table 3.1   Common risk factors for venous thromboembolism (VTE) in pregnancy

---

Patient factors

Age over 35 years

Obesity (BMI > 29 kg/m^2) in early pregnancy

Thrombophilia

Past history of VTE (especially if idiopathic or thrombophilia-associated)

Gross varicose veins

Significant current medical problem (e.g. nephrotic syndrome)

Current infection or inflammatory process (e.g. active inflammatory bowel disease
 or urinary tract infection)

Immobility (e.g. bed rest or lower limb fracture)

Paraplegia

Recent long-distance travel

Dehydration

Intravenous drug abuse

Ovarian hyperstimulation

Pregnancy/obstetric factors

Cesarean section particularly as an emergency in labor

Operative vaginal delivery

Major obstetric hemorrhage

Hyperemesis gravidarum

Pre-eclampsia

BMI, body mass index

An often overlooked area is the risk of VTE associated with ovarian stimulation for assisted conception therapy, where women are exposed not only to the pregnancy-associated risks of VTE but also to the effects of hyperestrogenism. Hyperstimulation is associated with procoagulant changes in the hemostatic and fibrinolytic systems[52]. As many as 6% of conceptions assisted by *in vitro* fertilization (IVF) can be complicated by hyperstimulation, and in 1–2% this can be severe. Venous and arterial thromboses are associated with hyperstimulation syndrome, although the overall rate of thrombosis in assisted conception is low. When venous thrombosis occurs, it is usually in the internal jugular vein, presenting with neck pain and swelling[53]. There may be an association with underlying thrombophilia, where the risk of VTE may be substantial. Indeed, to illustrate the extent of the risk, jugular vein thrombosis has been reported in a compound heterozygote for protein S deficiency and prothrombin G20210A despite therapeutic anticoagulation with a low-molecular-weight heparin, following IVF[54]. Thus, a risk assessment for thrombosis should be undertaken in women undergoing assisted conception therapy, and appropriate thromboprophylaxis, which may be therapeutic levels of anticoagulation, should be provided for those at high risk.

3.3 LONG-TERM MORBIDITY FROM PREGNANCY-ASSOCIATED VTE

A previous VTE is associated with an increased risk of future VTE. There is also a high risk of deep venous insufficiency developing: 80% of women with VTE develop post-thrombotic syndrome, and over 60% will have objectively confirmed deep venous insufficiency following a treated DVT[55]. Gestational DVT appears to carry the same risk of deep venous insufficiency as non-gestational DVT[55]. The risk of developing venous insufficiency after DVT is greater than with PTE: odds ratio (OR) 10.9 (95% confidence interval (CI) 4.2–28.0) for DVT compared with 3.8 (95% CI 1.2–12.3) after PTE[55]. This may be due to the clot clearing from the leg veins in those with PTE leading to less extensive damage to the deep venous system. This is a significant problem that obstetricians do not usually see, as these women present to dermatologists and vascular surgeons in later years. For example, Berqvist and colleagues[56] found that up to 21% of women with a treated DVT in pregnancy needed to use a compression bandage, and 6% had venous ulcers at a median time of follow-up of 10 years (Table 3.2). Historical data show rates for venous ulceration following untreated DVT to be 19–28% in follow-up periods ranging from 6 to 31 years[56].

Table 3.2 Subjective complaints in women followed up after pregnancy-associated deep vein thrombosis (DVT)[56]

	DVT during pregnancy (n = 61)	DVT during puerperium (n = 33)
Median follow-up time (years)	10 (range 7–21)	11 (range 7–26)
Leg swelling (%)	59	48
Varicose veins (%)	36	30
Discoloration (%)	28	27
Regular use of compression bandage (%)	21	3
Leg ulcer (%)	6.5	0

3.4 PATHOPHYSIOLOGY OF PREGNANCY-ASSOCIATED VTE

Virchow's triad of hypercoagulability, venous stasis and vascular damage occurs in the course of an uncomplicated pregnancy. First, there are increased levels of coagulation factors such as von Willebrand factor, factor VIII and fibrinogen, with the concentrations of some of these factors increasing by at least two-fold in the course of normal pregnancy. Almost 40% of pregnancies acquire resistance to the endogenous anticoagulant, activated protein C, and a reduction in protein S, the cofactor for protein C, is seen in normal pregnancy[24]. Fibrinolysis is physiologically impaired in pregnancy by increased levels of plasminogen activator inhibitors 1 and 2, the latter being produced by the placenta[57]. In the non-pregnant situation, high levels of factor VIII and resistance to activated protein C have been associated with an increased risk of VTE. Thus, these physiological changes in the hemostatic and fibrinolytic systems in pregnancy may explain, at least in part, the increased risk of thrombosis associated with pregnancy.

Second, relative venous stasis is a normal feature of pregnancy, and a substantial reduction in flow occurs by the end of the first trimester, progressing to around 50% reduction by 25–29 weeks' gestation, reaching a nadir at 36 weeks[58] and taking about 6 weeks to return to normal non-pregnant flow rates (Figure 3.3)[59].

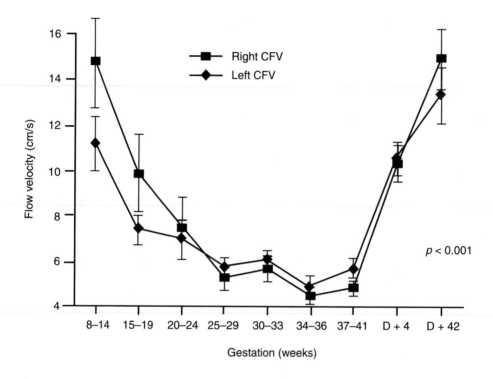

Figure 3.3   Changes in flow velocity (time-averaged mean velocity) in right and left common femoral veins (CFVs) in the course of pregnancy and the puerperium[58]. D, delivery + days

Third, some degree of endothelial damage to pelvic vessels appears inevitable as the veins are, at least to some degree, disturbed during the course of vaginal or abdominal delivery. Thus, the physiological changes of pregnancy and disturbance of the pelvic veins at delivery set the scene for the potential development of VTE.

Almost 90% of pregnancy-associated DVTs occur on the left side, in contrast to the non-pregnant situation where only 55% of DVTs occur on the left[51,60]. The underlying explanation is not clearly established, but it may reflect some compression of the left iliac vein by the right iliac artery and the ovarian artery, which cross the vein on the left side only. More than 70% of gestational DVTs are located in the ileofemoral region, compared with only around 9% in the non-pregnant situation, where calf vein DVTs are the most common. As ileofemoral DVTs are more likely to embolize and lead to PTE than calf vein thromboses, this is an important difference between gestational and non-gestational DVT. Lower abdominal pain can be a presenting feature of DVT in pregnancy. This may be due to the opening up of a periovarian collateral venous circulation, or thrombosis extending into the pelvic veins. This pain is usually associated with a mild fever and leukocytosis, which are well recognized features of venous thrombosis. This presentation may cause diagnostic confusion, and DVT may be mistaken for other intra-abdominal problems such as appendicitis. Thus, it is important to consider DVT as a possible diagnosis in a woman presenting with these features in pregnancy, especially as the clinical diagnosis of DVT is entirely unreliable.

3.5 THROMBOPHILIA AND PREGNANCY-ASSOCIATED VENOUS THROMBOSIS

One or more heritable or acquired thrombophilias are now found in at least 50% of cases of VTE in pregnancy. The main heritable thrombophilias recognized currently include deficiencies of the endogenous anticoagulant proteins, antithrombin, protein C and protein S, and abnormalities of procoagulants, particularly factor V Leiden and the so called prothrombin gene variant (prothrombin 20210A).

Deficiencies of antithrombin, protein C and protein S, where the major components of the body's endogenous anticoagulant system are defective or deficient owing to quantitative or qualitative defects, are

Table 3.3   Prevalence rates for congenital thrombophilia in European populations

Thrombophilic defect	Prevalance (%)
Antithrombin deficiency	0.25–0.55
Protein C deficiency	0.20–0.33
Factor V Leiden heterozygotes	2–7
Prothrombin 20210A heterozygotes	2
MTHFR C677T homozygotes	10

MTHFR, methylene-tetrahydrofolate reductase

uncommon (Table 3.3). They have a combined prevalence of less than 1%[61], although it should be noted that the prevalence of protein S deficiency is not well established. Investigation of gestational VTE will reveal one of these defects in fewer than 10% of cases.

Factor V Leiden is functionally manifest as resistance to activated protein C, the endogenous anticoagulant that inactivates factor Va and factor VIIIa by proteolytic cleavage. Resistance is due to a single point mutation in the factor V gene. This alteration in factor V at the cleavage site (Arg506) results in a potentially hypercoagulable effect, as the activated factor V cannot be broken down by activated protein C. Factor V Leiden occurs in 2–7% in Western European populations (Table 3.3)[61], and will usually be identified in 20–40% of women with a gestational (or non-gestational) VTE[62]. Activated protein C resistance is acquired in around 40% of pregnancies in the absence of factor V Leiden[24], probably due to gestational increases in factor V and factor VIII. Such acquired changes are relevant, as outwith pregnancy, high levels of factor VIII and activated protein C resistance, not associated with factor V Leiden, are both independently associated with an increase in risk of VTE. Activated protein C resistance can also be seen with other thrombophilic problems such as antiphospholipid antibody syndrome, and genetic abnormalities other than factor V Leiden (FV) such as factor V Cambridge or the HR2 haplotype. Although defects such as FV Cambridge are uncommon, the HR2 haplotype is relatively common, and has been reported to carry an excess risk of VTE in patients with a high risk profile (OR 1.8, 95% CI 1.1–2.8), including pregnancy[63]. It is of interest that, although factor V Leiden is associated with an increase in risk of VTE, this is largely due to DVT. Outwith pregnancy, the prevalence of underlying factor V Leiden in PTE is around half that for DVT[64]. This varies from other thrombophilias such as prothrombin G20210A, where there is no difference in the underlying prevalence between DVT and PTE. The mechanism is not clear. It has been proposed that factor V Leiden is associated with a more adherent and stable thrombus, possibly owing to increased local thrombin generation, thus reducing the likelihood of embolization. Whether this applies in pregnancy to women with factor V Leiden is not yet clear.

Prothrombin G20210A, the prothrombin gene variant, occurs in the heterozygous form in about 2% of Western European populations. This genotype is expressed as elevated plasma prothrombin (factor II, FII) levels. It appears to increase the risk of venous thrombosis three-fold[65].

Prothrombin (FII) G20210A can be found in around 6% of patients with VTE, and has been reported in almost 20% of those with a strong family history of VTE[65]. Gestational VTE has been linked to this genotype[66,67].

It is noteworthy that the FV Leiden and prothrombin G20210A genotypes do not occur with similar frequencies in all populations. For example, in the Taiwan Chinese, factor V Leiden and prothrombin G20210A were found in only 0.2% and 0.2% of the population compared with 4.8% and 1.2%, respectively, in a control population of Newfoundlanders[68].

Hyperhomocysteinemia has been linked to VTE in the non-pregnant situation[69]. Hyperhomocysteinemia can be associated with homozygosity for a variant of the methylene-tetrahydrofolate reductase gene (MTHFR C677T), sometimes called the thermolabile variant. This genotype itself is not directly linked to venous thrombosis, but predisposes to arterial and venous thrombosis where there is concomitant vitamin-B deficiency. Around 10% of individuals in Western European populations are homozygous for this common genetic variant. However, such homozygotes do not appear to be at increased risk of pregnancy related VTE[66,70,71]. The reason for this is unclear, but, as clinical events in homozygotes are likely to reflect the interaction of the genotype with a relative deficiency of B vitamins such as folic acid, the absence of an association of this genotype with gestational VTE may reflect the pregnancy related physiological reduction in homocysteine levels and/or the effects of folic acid supplements that are now taken widely by women in pregnancy for the prevention of neural tube defects.

Potentially, thrombophilic abnormalities are common, affecting at least 15% of Western populations[72,73], and underlie around 50% of gestational VTEs. Yet only around one in 1000 pregnancies is complicated by a clinical VTE. Thus, thrombophilia alone, even in conjunction with the gestational changes in hemostatic and fibrinolytic systems and reduced venous flow, does not invariably lead to thrombosis. This is because clinical thrombosis in women with thrombophilia is a multicausal event, resulting from the interaction between congenital and acquired risk factors[73]. The likelihood of thrombosis depends on the thrombophilia, whether more than one thrombophilia is present, whether previous VTEs have occurred and additional risk factors such as obesity.

It is important to consider the level of risk for thrombosis during pregnancy in women with thrombophilia, to guide the need for thromboprophylaxis. Much of our existing knowledge comes from observational studies of symptomatic thrombophilic kindred. This will overestimate the risk for previously asymptomatic women with thrombophilia, and also for asymptomatic families where a thrombophilia has been identified coincidentally. For example, initial estimates for the risk of gestational VTE without anticoagulant therapy ranged from 32 to 60% in antithrombin-deficient women[61,74–76]. Estimates for the risk of gestational thrombosis vary between 3 and 10% for protein C deficiency and 0 and 6% for protein S deficiency during pregnancy, rising to 7–19% and 7–22%, respectively, for protein C deficiency and protein S deficiency postpartum[61,74–76]. Factor V Leiden has been reported in up to 46% of women investigated for gestational VTE[77]. It must be recognized that these data reflect the prevalence in symptomatic women, and do not provide information on the risk of thrombosis in previously asymptomatic women with thrombophilias. Several recent studies have provided estimates for the risk of gestational thrombosis in the more common thrombophilias. Gerhardt and colleagues[71] assessed 119 women with thromboembolism in pregnancy and 233 controls for the presence of thrombophilia. The relative risk for thrombosis in pregnancy after adjusting for other key variables was 6.9 (95% CI 3.3–15.2) with factor V Leiden, 9.5 (95% CI 2.1–66.7) with prothrombin G20210A and 10.4 (95% CI 2.2–62.5) for antithrombin deficiency. Combined defects substantially increase risk, with an OR estimated at 107 for the combination of factor V Leiden and prothrombin G20210A. Additional risk factors such as obesity were present in 25% of cases compared with 11% of controls. Women with recurrent events were more likely to have an underlying combined thrombophilia. This study also provided a positive predictive value for each thrombophilia, assuming an underlying rate of venous thromboembolism of 0.66/1000 pregnancies, consistent with estimates from Western populations[72]. These values were 1 : 500 for factor V Leiden, 1 : 200 for prothrombin 20210A and 4.6 : 100 for these defects combined. Homozygotes for defects such as factor V Leiden also have a greater level of risk than heterozygotes. For example, the absolute risk of VTE with homozygous factor V Leiden has been reported to be 9.5% (95% CI 6–14%)[78]. A retrospective study of 72 000 pregnancies, where women with venous thrombosis were assessed for thrombophilia[51] and where the underlying prevalence of these defects in the population was known, found that the risk of thrombosis was 1 : 437 for factor V Leiden, 1 : 113 for protein C deficiency, 1 : 2.8 for type 1 (quantitative) antithrombin deficiency and 1 : 42 for type 2 (qualitative) antithrombin deficiency. This study was extended[66], and reported an odds ratio of 4.4 (95% CI 1.2–16) for prothrombin G20210A, 4.5 (95% CI 2.1–14.5) for factor V Leiden, 282 (95% CI 31–2532) for antithrombin deficiency type 1 (quantitative deficiency) and 28 (95% CI 5.5–142) for antithrombin deficiency type 2 (qualitative deficiency) (Table 3.4). More recently, Martinelli and

Table 3.4   Risk of venous thromboembolism (VTE) in pregnancy with thrombophilia

Thrombophilic defect	Odds ratio (95% CI) for VTE in pregnancy*	Relative risk (95% CI) for VTE in pregnancy†	Relative risk (95% CI) for VTE in pregnancy or puerperium**
AT deficiency Type 1 (quantitative deficiency)	282 (31–2532)	NA	NA
AT deficiency Type 2 (qualitative deficiency)	28 (5.5–142)	NA	NA
AT deficiency (activity < 80%)	NA	10.4 (2.2–62.5)	NA
FV Leiden heterozygotes	4.5 (2.1–14.5)	6.9 (3.3–15.2)	8.7 (3.4–22.5)
Prothrombin 20210A heterozygotes	4.4 (1.2–16)	9.5 (2.1–66.7)	1.8 (0.6–5.4)
MTHFR C677T homozygotes	0.45 (0.13–1.58)	no increase in risk (RR not reported)	NA
Any thrombophilia	NA	NA	9.0 (4.7–17.1)
Antithrombin, protein C or protein S deficiency (not adjusted for parity)	NA	NA	13.1 (5.0–34.5)

*Based on a retrospective study of 93 000 pregnancies where odds ratios were calculated by screening women with VTE in pregnancy for thrombophilia and relating this to the known prevalence of these defects in the population[66]; †based on a study of 119 women with thromboembolism in pregnancy and 233 controls for the presence of congenital thrombophilia[71]: relative risk (RR) calculated after logistic regression to adjust for age, body mass index, oral contraceptive use, protein C and S activity, factor V Leiden, prothrombin G20210A, methylene-tetrahydrofolate reductase (MTHFR) 677TT and antithrombin (AT) activity; **based on a case–control study of 119 cases who had a first episode of objectively confirmed VTE in pregnancy or the puerperium and 232 controls: relative risk adjusted for parity, no difference between relative risk in pregnancy or puerperium[79]; NA, not available associates[79] reported a case–control study of 119 women with a first episode of VTE during pregnancy or the puerperium. The unadjusted relative risk for VTE was 10.6 (95% CI 5.6–20.4) for heterozygotes of factor V Leiden, 2.9 (95% CI 1.0–8.6) for prothrombin G20210A heterozygotes and 13.1 (95% CI 5.0–34.2) for protein C, protein S and antithrombin deficiency grouped together (Table 3.4). These data are valuable in evaluating risk and advising women whether to use thromboprophylaxis in pregnancy.

3.6 THROMBOPHILIA AND ADVERSE PREGNANCY OUTCOME

Thrombophilias are not only associated with an increased risk of VTE, but also with pregnancy complications. In particular, there is good evidence linking antiphospholipid antibody syndrome, which is associated with increased thrombin generation[80], to recurrent miscarriage. The importance of procoagulant changes in the pathophysiology of recurrent miscarriage associated with antiphospholipid antibody syndrome is emphasized by the success of treatment with heparin and low-dose aspirin, which substantially reduces the risk of miscarriage[81], although a recent randomized trial has reported no difference in outcome between women with recurrent miscarriage treated with low-dose aspirin alone and those treated with low-dose aspirin and heparin in combination[82]. This antithrombotic therapy is essentially the only successful medical intervention in the treatment of miscarriage. A recent meta-analysis reported that combination therapy with aspirin and heparin may reduce pregnancy loss by 54% in women with antiphospholipid antibody syndrome[83]. Such associations led to the study of heritable thrombophilia and pregnancy complications that might be associated with thrombotic damage to the placenta.

One early cohort study of women with thrombophilia reviewed their pregnancy outcome. This was carried out by the European prospective cohort study on thrombophilia (EPCOT)[84]. The thrombophilic disorders assessed were antithrombin, protein C and protein S deficiencies and factor V Leiden. In view of the possibility that symptomatic thrombophilia may be related to multigenic problems, patients with combined defects were also assessed. The data were compared with those for a healthy control population. Overall, there was an increased risk of fetal loss (OR 1.35, 95% CI 1.01–1.82) and stillbirth

(OR 3.6, 95% CI 1.4–9.4). However, the risk of miscarriage was not significantly increased (OR 1.27, 95% CI 0.94–1.71). A further retrospective study on antithrombin, protein C and protein S deficiency found a higher incidence of pregnancy loss in antithrombin, protein C and protein S deficiency with an OR of 2.0 (95% CI 1.2–3.3) for all deficiencies combined[85]. A large number of case–control studies have now evaluated associations between thrombophilia and pregnancy loss[72,86–92]. Although there are inconsistencies, these studies suggest a possible association between factor V Leiden and recurrent early fetal loss, with a much clearer association with late fetal loss. Homozygosity for MTHFR C677T, present in around 10% of Europeans and associated with hyperhomocysteinemia, has also been evaluated in the context of adverse pregnancy outcomes. However, overall, the evidence does not favor an association. This might reflect the fact that hyperhomocysteinemia associated with MTHFR C677T homozygotes requires an interaction of acquired dietary factors with the genotype. The lack of association might also reflect the physiological fall in homocysteine levels seen in normal pregnancy, or the effects of folic acid supplements that are widely used in pregnancy to prevent neural tube defects.

A further hypercoagulable state that is acquired is the presence of circulating procoagulant microparticles, which is associated with several prothrombotic conditions[93]. These microparticles are derived from the cell membrane, being released following cell activation when there is remodelling of the membrane leading to externalization of the aminophospholipids, such as phosphotidylserine, in the plasma membrane. These particles can enhance tissue factor activity (which is closely linked to the presence of phosphotidylserine), provide a catalytic surface for the assembly of procoagulant enzyme complexes and activate platelets[93]. Laude and colleagues[94] measured these microparticles outwith pregnancy in women with a history of pregnancy loss, and compared results with those for controls. Prothrombotic microparticle levels above the upper limit of normal were found in 59% of the recurrent miscarriage group and in 48% of the late fetal loss group. The association with fetal loss could be due to the vulnerability of the trophoblast to prothrombotic attack by these particles.

The association between various hypercoagulable states and pregnancy loss raises some interesting questions. Perhaps the consideration of hypercoagulable states underlying pregnancy loss has been too specific. There are associations with various heritable and acquired thrombophilias. Thus, hypercoagulable states associated with increased thrombin generation in general, rather than acquired or heritable thrombophilia in particular, may be responsible for pregnancy loss. From a therapeutic perspective, this concept should lead to the assessment of intervention with antithrombotic therapy; there is some evidence from small studies that this may be effective[86], and several randomized trials of low-molecular-weight heparin are ongoing in this area. Their results are awaited with interest and will inform our management of recurrent pregnancy loss.

The widespread vascular damage of pre-eclampsia is associated with endothelial dysfunction, enhanced coagulation and fibrin deposition which play a role in the vascular insult, leading to end-organ damage such as in the kidney, brain and placenta. Intrauterine growth restriction (IUGR) is associated with placental infarction on the maternal side. Thus, thrombophilias could predispose a woman to these pregnancy complications.

There have been reports of both heritable and acquired thrombophilias being associated with pre-eclampsia. Case–control studies have reported a 2–5-fold increased carrier rate for FV Leiden (or abnormal activated protein C (APC) resistance) in subjects with a history of pre-eclampsia[72,86,95]. Kupferminc and associates[95] reported ORs for developing pre-eclampsia, stillbirth, IUGR or abruption collectively of 3.7 (95% CI 1.5–9.0) for FV Leiden and 3.9 (95% CI 1.1–14.6) for prothrombin 20210A. The degree of acquired aPC resistance in pregnancy, in FV Leiden-negative subjects, has also been associated with around a three-fold risk of pre-eclampsia[96].

A recent systematic review[97] has also evaluated these relationships. This review reported a significant association between pre-eclampsia and factor V Leiden heterozygotes and homozygotes, prothrombin G20210A heterozygotes, MTHFR C677T homozygotes and protein C and S deficiency[97]. With regard to IUGR, this review reported, on meta-analysis, an association between IUGR and heterozygotes for prothrombin G20210A, homozygotes for MTHFR C677T, protein S deficiency and anticardiolipin antibodies[97]. Other pregnancy complications were also linked to thrombophilic defects; for example, both abruption and stillbirth had a positive association with factor V Leiden and anticardiolipin antibodies. However, a more recent meta-analysis published in conjunction with a large population-based study did not find an association between pre-eclampsia and factor V Leiden, prothrombin

G20210A, MTHFR C677T or platelet collagen receptor, α2β1C807T, in a population of 404 women with a history of pre-eclampsia compared with 303 with gestational hypertension and 164 controls[98]. This meta-analysis of studies of pre-eclampsia and thrombophilia, with appropriate inclusion criteria, reported that there was no overall association between pre-eclampsia and factor V Leiden, prothrombin G20210A and MTHFR C677T homozygotes. However, when the analysis was restricted to severe pre-eclampsia, there was a significant association with factor V Leiden and with MTHFR C677T homozygotes, with pooled ORs of 2.84 (95% CI 1.95–4.14) and 1.5 (95% CI 1.02–2.23), respectively. No association was found between severe pre-eclampsia and prothrombin G20210A. The reasons underlying these differences in results with regard to the association between thrombophilia and pregnancy complications are unclear. They may reflect different diagnostic criteria, small sample size and reporting bias, as many studies had relatively low levels of heterozygosity for factor V Leiden in the control groups studied. None the less, these data suggest that prothrombotic genotypes may not be causative factors for pre-eclampsia, but may be linked to the severity of disease expression once the condition arises, presumably by enhancing the coagulation response associated with these conditions.

A recent large case–control study has also cast doubt on the association between IUGR and thrombophilia[99]. This study of 493 newborns with IUGR and 472 controls found no increase in risk of IUGR among mothers carrying MTHFR C677T, factor V Leiden or prothrombin G20210A, with ORs of 1.55 (95% CI 0.83–2.90), 1.18 (95% CI 0.54–2.35) and 0.92 (95% CI 0.36–2.35), respectively[99]. Even when the birth weight centile was reduced to the 5th centile and the analysis repeated, there was no relationship, suggesting that, in contrast to pre-eclampsia, there is no relationship to disease severity. However, there was an association between MTHFR C677T homozygotes and IUGR in the subgroup of mothers not taking vitamin supplements (OR 12.3, 95% CI 1.2–126.2). Thus, the lack of association between IUGR and MTHFR C677T homozygotes may reflect the widespread use of multivitamin preparations containing folic acid in pregnancy, which could influence homocysteine levels, and emphasizes the need for consideration of plasma homocysteine rather than the MTHFR genotype alone. Thus, the interaction between genes and environment is likely to be important in clinical manifestations of thrombophilias. In addition, this study reported that there was no association with the fetal genotype for thrombophilia; indeed, homozygosity in the fetus for MTHFR C677T was associated with a reduced risk of IUGR (OR 0.52, 95% CI 0.29–0.94)[99]. The differences between this study and previous reports are first, the size, and, second, the possibility of selection bias for subjects as the prevalence of various polymorphisms was similar in the control populations in previous studies.

Defects in fibrinolysis can also play a role. The hypofibrinolytic 4G/4G mutation of the plasminogen activator inhibitor (PAI-1) gene is associated with higher PAI-1 levels than those found in individuals with the 5G/5G genotype. 4G/5G polymorphisms have been linked with arterial disease, especially coronary heart disease, and venous thrombosis. This genotype has been assessed as a possible factor contributing to pregnancy complications (severe pre-eclampsia, placental abruption, IUGR and stillbirth). In a study of 94 women with a previous pregnancy complication and 95 controls, the women who had had pregnancy complications were more likely than controls to be homozygotes for the 4G mutation (32% vs. 19%), giving an OR of 2.0 (95% CI 1.02–3.9). However, many cases also carried the factor V Leiden gene. None the less, mutations in the PAI-1 gene were independently associated with obstetric complications (OR 1.56, 95% CI 1.005–2.43). This study also reported that 76% of cases had some form of thrombophilia or hypofibrinolysis, compared with 37% of controls, so emphasizing the association between thrombophilic defects, particularly when found in combination, and adverse pregnancy outcome[100]. Again, however, there are inconsistencies in the published data, as Morrison and co-workers[98] did not find an association with pre-eclampsia in heterozygotes for the 4G mutation (4G/5G).

There are also mutations in the coagulation system that appear to protect against thrombotic events. A G-to-T point mutation in exon 2 of the factor XIII (FXIII) A-subunit gene results in a leucine rather than valine at amino acid position 34 of the factor XIII molecule. This mutation has been associated with a reduced risk of both arterial and venous thrombosis. A recent study assessed whether this might protect against pre-eclampsia. In subjects heterozygous for the T genotype (GT), the relative risk of pre-eclampsia was 0.7 (95% CI 0.4–1.1) when compared with the GG genotype. For subjects homozygous for the T allele, the relative risk for pre-eclampsia was 0.8 (95% CI 0.3–2.1) when compared with the GG genotype. The risk associated with the T allele in the heterozygous and homozygous forms versus the GG genotype was 0.7 (95% CI 0.4–1.1). Thus, this mutation's protective effect on thrombotic events does not extend to protection against pre-eclampsia, at least not to the magnitude of that reported in other thrombotic disease[101].

3.7 SCREENING FOR CONGENITAL THROMBOPHILIA IN PREGNANCY

At present there is no evidence to support universal screening for thrombophilia in pregnancy, for the prevention of either VTE or pregnancy complications. The natural history of many of these thrombophilias, particularly in asymptomatic kindred, is not yet established, appropriate intervention is unclear and cost-effectiveness is not established. A recent study has shown that universal screening for factor V Leiden in pregnancy is not cost-effective (Table 3.5)[102]. Selective screening of women with VTE in pregnancy or who have a personal or family history of, ideally objectively confirmed, VTE may be of value, as around 50% of such women will have a heritable thrombophilia. There is consensus that women with a personal history of VTE and an underlying thrombophilia should receive thromboprophylaxis with low-molecular-weight heparin (LMWH) during pregnancy and with LMWH or coumarin in the puerperium[103]. Screening for thrombophilia in patients with problems such as recurrent miscarriage, intrauterine death, IUGR and pre-eclampsia, which may all be associated with an underlying thrombophilia and therefore risk of VTE, should also be considered[72]. However, apart from recurrent miscarriage associated with antiphospholipid antibody syndrome, effective intervention is not established. None the less, if these women have a thrombophilia that is symptomatic in relation to a pregnancy complication, they may also be at risk of venous thrombosis owing to the presence of multiple risk factors including a thrombophilia or a severe thrombophilia such as antithrombin deficiency, conditions that would themselves merit specific thromboprophylaxis. As in any screening situation, appropriate counselling should be offered.

Thrombophilia screening is of limited value in women with acute VTE. However, at the very least this should include assessing the woman for a family history of thrombosis (Table 3.6). A laboratory

Table 3.5 Cost-effectiveness of screening for factor V (FV) Leiden in pregnancy[102]. Costs are given in £

	No screening (n = 967)	Selective screening (n = 113)	Universal screening (n = 967)
Cost of screening for mutation	0	1 305.31	11 543.29
Cost of prophylactic postpartum LMWH for those positive for FV Leiden	0	595.48	5 959.80
Cost of prophylactic LMWH (from 12–40 weeks' gestation) for those positive for FV Leiden	0	2 774.94	27 787.20
Averted costs of treating vascular events (assumes 50% reduction with prophylaxis)	0	908.13	5448.81
Net cost of treatment for whole cohort	158 013.4	157 105.3	152 566.6
Total cost of management strategy	158 013.4	161 781.0	197 856.9
Number identified with FV Leiden	0	3	30
Number with complications associated with FV Leiden	87	1	6
Events prevented by screening (assumes 50% reduction with prophylaxis)	0	0.5	3

LMWH, low-molecular-weight heparin

Table 3.6 Thrombophilia screening

APTT (may identify anticardiolipin antibodies)
Prothrombin time (aids interpretation of low protein C or S)
Thrombin time (can identify dysfibrinogenemia or heparin contamination)

Activated protein C resistance (N.B. genetic testing for factor V Leiden is only required where there is evidence of activated protein C (aPC) resistance on the modified test for aPC resistance that predilutes the test sample with factor V-deficient plasma)

Protein C deficiency
Protein S deficiency
Antithrombin deficiency
Prothrombin 20210A mutation
Lupus anticoagulant
Anticardiolipin antibodies (IgG and IgM)

APTT, activated partial thromboplastin time; Ig, immunoglobulin

40

assessment (ideally prior to anticoagulant therapy) can be considered, although it is ideal to delay full laboratory screening until 1 month after anticoagulation has been discontinued. The results of a thrombophilia screen will not usually influence the diagnosis or the immediate management of acute VTE; however, it may influence the duration and intensity of anticoagulation, such as when antithrombin deficiency is identified in pregnancy. It is important to be aware of the effects of pregnancy and thrombus on the results of a thrombophilia screen, and thrombophilia screens taken in pregnancy must be interpreted by clinicians with specific expertise in the area. For example, protein S levels fall in normal pregnancy, making it virtually impossible to make a diagnosis of protein S deficiency during pregnancy. Activated protein C resistance occurs in around 40% of pregnancies, and anticardiolipin antibodies can also influence the result of this test. Antithrombin may be reduced when a thrombus is present. Other factors can also influence the results of a thrombophilia screen; for example, in nephrotic syndrome antithrombin levels are reduced, and in liver disease proteins C and S will be reduced. Clearly, genotyping for factor V Leiden and prothrombin G20210A will not be influenced by pregnancy or current thrombosis. It is important, therefore, that thrombophilia screens be interpreted by clinicians with specific expertise.

3.8 DIAGNOSIS OF VTE IN PREGNANCY

The clinical features of DVT include leg pain or discomfort (especially on the left), swelling, tenderness, increased temperature and edema, lower abdominal pain, mild pyrexia and elevated white cell count. Features suggestive of PTE include dyspnea, collapse, chest pain, hemoptysis, faintness, raised jugular venous pressure and focal signs in the chest, sometimes combined with the symptoms and signs of DVT. Just as in the non-pregnant, the clinical diagnosis of VTE during pregnancy is unreliable, particularly as problems such as leg swelling and discomfort are common features of normal pregnancy. In a study of consecutive pregnant women presenting with a clinical suspicion of DVT, the diagnosis was confirmed in fewer than 10%[103]. This compares with about 25% of diagnoses being confirmed in the non-pregnant situation[104,105]. Around 30% of patients presenting with possible PTE outwith pregnancy have the diagnosis confirmed[106,107], but the number of positive results following investigation appears to be substantially lower in pregnancy[103], possibly because of a low threshold for investigation. Objective diagnosis of VTE in pregnancy is therefore essential, as failure to identify a VTE will endanger the mother while unnecessary treatment will expose her to the hazards of therapeutic anticoagulation. Such treatment may also label her as having had a VTE, a factor that will significantly alter her future health care with regard to contraception, thromboprophylaxis in future pregnancies and hormone replacement therapy in later life.

Real-time or Duplex ultrasound venography is the main diagnostic tool[108] for DVT. If DVT is confirmed, anticoagulant treatment should be commenced or continued. In non-pregnant subjects, the pre-test clinical probability of DVT modifies both the positive predictive value and the negative predictive value of objective diagnostic tests[109,110]. Applying this to pregnancy, a negative ultrasound result with a low level of clinical suspicion suggests that anticoagulant treatment can be discontinued or withheld. With a negative ultrasound report and a high level of clinical suspicion, the woman should be anticoagulated and ultrasound repeated in 1 week, or alternative imaging techniques such as X-ray venography or magnetic resonance imaging (MRI) should be considered. If repeat testing is negative, anticoagulant treatment should be discontinued[111] (Table 3.7).

Where PTE is suspected, both a ventilation/perfusion (V/Q) lung scan and bilateral duplex ultrasound leg examinations should ideally be performed. Outwith pregnancy, a normal ventilation perfusion scan has a negative predictive value of over 99% and a high-probability lung scan has a positive predictive value of over 85%. Where there is a strong clinical suspicion of PTE, the positive predictive value of a high-probability lung scan increases to over 95%, but with low clinical probability decreases to under 60%. The greatest diagnostic problem is when the V/Q scan is in the medium range. In practical terms, when the V/Q scan reports a 'medium' or 'high' probability of PTE, or where there is a 'low' probability of PTE on V/Q scan but positive ultrasound for DVT, anticoagulant treatment should be continued. When a V/Q scan reports a low risk of PTE and there are negative leg ultrasound examinations, yet there remains a high level of clinical suspicion, anticoagulant treatment should continue with repeat testing in 1 week (V/Q scan and leg ultrasound examination), or alternative imaging techniques such as pulmonary angiography, MRI or helical computerized tomography (CT)

Table 3.7   Suggested treatment following results of investigations for gestational venous thromboembolism (VTE)

Suspected DVT: a negative ultrasound venography result with a low level of clinical suspicion	anticoagulant treatment can be discontinued or withheld
Suspected DVT: a negative ultrasound venography report and a high level of clinical suspicion	the woman should be anticoagulated and the ultrasound repeated in 1 week or X-ray venography should be considered. If repeat testing is negative, anticoagulant treatment should be discontinued
Suspected DVT: positive ultrasound examination	start or continue anticoagulant treatment
Suspected PTE: the V/Q scan reports a 'medium' or 'high' probability of PTE	anticoagulant treatment should be continued
Suspected PTE: a 'low' probability of PTE on V/Q scan but positive ultrasound venography for DVT	anticoagulant treatment should be continued
Suspected PTE: a V/Q scan reports a low probability of PTE and there are negative leg ultrasound venography examinations, yet there is a high level of clinical suspicion	anticoagulant treatment should continue with repeat testing in 1 week (V/Q scan and leg ultrasound venography examination) or alternative imaging technique such as helical CT, echocardiography or MRI employed
Suspected PTE: a V/Q scan reports a low probability of PTE and there are negative leg ultrasound venography examinations, and there is a low level of clinical suspicion	discontinue anticoagulation

DVT, deep vein thrombosis; PTE, pulmonary thromboembolism; V/Q, ventilation/perfusion; CT, computerized tomography; MRI, magnetic resonance imaging

should be employed[111]. Similarly, if the chest X-ray has abnormalities which lead to difficulties in the diagnosis of PTE using V/Q scanning, then alternative imaging techniques are warranted. Helical CT scanning is likely to be of particular value, and as the test becomes more widely available will threaten the place of V/Q scans in the diagnosis of PTE. Helical CT can rapidly image the whole thorax within the time of a single breath hold, with good visualization of the pulmonary arterial tree down to the level of the segmental arteries; technical advances are likely to allow even greater resolution and faster image acquisition times. It can sometimes be useful to employ echocardiography of the right heart, particularly when performed transesophageally, where PTE is suspected. This may allow direct visualization of a thrombus in the pulmonary arteries or right heart. Indirect signs of PTE include a dilated hypokinetic right ventricle, tricuspid regurgitation and high pulmonary artery pressures as measured with Doppler ultrasound. It must be emphasized that the radiation dose from investigations such as V/Q scanning, chest X-ray and even limited venography is modest[112], and considered to pose a negligible risk to the fetus particularly when set in the context of the risk from PTE. For example, the radiation dose from a chest X-ray is less than that obtained over 10 days from background radiation or 20 h of air travel. Thus, objective diagnostic testing should not be withheld because of concern regarding fetal radiation exposure.

D-dimer is now used as a screening test for VTE in the non-pregnant where it has a high negative predictive value[108], i.e. a low level of D-dimer suggests the absence of VTE and further objective tests are not performed, while an increased level of D-dimer leads to an objective diagnostic test for VTE. In pregnancy, D-dimer can be increased owing to the physiological changes in the coagulation system, and particularly if there is a concomitant problem such as pre-eclampsia or antepartum hemorrhage. Thus, a 'positive' D-dimer test in pregnancy is not necessarily consistent with VTE, and objective diagnostic testing is required. However, a low level of D-dimer in pregnancy is likely, as in the non-pregnant, to suggest that there is no VTE. None the less, there is limited information on the efficacy and safety of D-dimer screening for VTE in pregnancy, and, until more information is available, firm guidance cannot be given.

3.9 ANTITHROMBOTIC THERAPY IN PREGNANCY

Coumarins

Treatment and prophylaxis of gestational VTE center on the use of unfractionated heparin (UFH) or LMWH, owing to the fetal hazards of coumarins[113]. Although coumarins such as warfarin are not secreted in breast milk in clinically significant amounts and are therefore safe to use during lactation, they cross the placenta and are known teratogens. Coumarin embryopathy (consisting of mid-face hypoplasia, stippled chondral calcification, scoliosis, short proximal limbs and short phalanges) may occur with exposure to the drug between 6 and 9 weeks' gestation. The incidence of this condition has been estimated at around 5%[113]. This problem is potentially preventable by substitution of heparin for warfarin during the first trimester. The risk of embryopathy may be dose-dependent, as an increased risk has been reported when the dose of warfarin is greater than 5 mg/day[114]. In addition to warfarin embryopathy, there is the possibility of problems arising due to fetal bleeding. As the fetal liver is immature and fetal levels of vitamin K-dependent coagulation factors low, maternal warfarin therapy maintained in the therapeutic range is likely to be associated with excessive anticoagulation and, therefore, potential hemorrhagic complications in the fetus. Coumarin should therefore be avoided beyond 36 weeks' gestation[113,115] because of the excessive hemorrhagic risk to both mother and fetus. In addition, it should be noted that recent data show that prenatal exposure to coumarins is associated with an increased risk of disturbance in development, manifest as minor neurological dysfunction or a low intelligence quotient in school-age children, with a relative risk of 7.6 for two or more of these minor abnormalities[116].

Heparins

Neither UFH[117] nor LMWH cross the placenta[118,119], as determined by measuring anti-Xa activity in fetal blood, and there is no evidence of teratogenesis or risk of fetal hemorrhage. On systematic review, LMWHs appear to be safe for the fetus[120]. Heparins are not secreted in breast milk and can be used during breast-feeding. Prolonged use of UFH is associated with symptomatic osteoporosis, with around a 2% incidence of osteoporotic fractures, allergy and heparin-induced thrombocytopenia[121]. However, LMWH appears to have a substantially lower risk of osteoporosis. A recent randomized trial of UFH or dalteparin for thromboprophylaxis in pregnancy measured bone mineral density in the lumbar spine for up to 3 years after delivery[122]. Bone density did not differ between healthy controls and the dalteparin group, but was significantly lower in the UFH group when compared with both controls and dalteparin-treated women. Multiple logistic regression found that the type of heparin therapy was the only independent factor associated with reduced bone mass. Heparin-induced thrombocytopenia is uncommon, but none the less important. It is an idiosyncratic immune reaction associated with extensive venous thrombosis. It usually occurs between 5 and 15 days after starting heparin. The risk is around 1–3% with UFH and is substantially lower, indeed negligible, with LMWH[123]. Allergic reactions usually take the form of itchy, erythematous lesions at the injection sites. Changing the heparin preparation may be helpful, but cross-reactivity can occur. Allergic reactions should be distinguished from faulty injection technique with associated bruising. LMWH is now the heparin of choice in pregnancy because of a better side-effect profile, good safety record for mother and fetus and convenient once-daily dosing for prophylaxis[120,124–129]. Almost 1500 cases of prophylaxis or treatment of VTE in pregnancy with enoxaparin and dalteparin, the two most commonly reported LMWHs in pregnancy, have now been reported in the literature, and the risk of recurrent VTE is around 1.2% and of symptomatic osteoporotic fracture 0.007% (unpublished data).

Hirudin, a direct thrombin inhibitor, is used in the non-pregnant for treatment of heparin-induced thrombocytopenia, and is also used for postoperative prophylaxis. As it crosses the placenta, it should not be used in pregnancy. It has been used in a lactating mother because of heparin-induced thrombocytopenia and hirudin was not detectable in breast milk[130].

Other antithrombotic therapies

Dextran has been used for peripartum thromboprophylaxis, particularly during Cesarean section. It has a significant risk of anaphylactic and anaphylactoid reactions. There is a risk of maternal anaphylactoid reactions which have been associated with uterine hypertonus, profound fetal distress and a high incidence of fetal death or profound neurological damage[131]. Thus, dextran should be avoided in pregnancy.

Graduated elastic compression stockings are effective in the non-pregnant and, in view of the pregnancy-related changes in the venous system, could be of value in pregnancy. They may act by preventing overdistension of veins, so preventing endothelial damage and exposure of subendothelial collagen[132]. They can also be employed in acute DVT. Other mechanical techniques such as intermittent pneumatic compression are of value during Cesarean section and immediately postpartum for prophylaxis.

Aspirin has been found in meta-analysis to have a beneficial effect in the prevention of DVT. Its effectiveness for VTE prophylaxis in pregnancy, in comparison with heparin, remains to be established, but it is likely to offer some benefit. Its effectiveness is likely to be less than that of heparin and LMWH[133]. In women who are unable to take heparin or in whom the balance of risk is not considered sufficient to merit heparin, it may be useful. Low-dose (60–75 mg daily) aspirin is not associated with adverse pregnancy outcome in the second and third trimesters[134,135].

3.10 MANAGEMENT OF ACUTE GESTATIONAL VTE

When a VTE is suspected, treatment with UFH or LMWH should be given until the diagnosis is excluded by objective testing, unless anticoagulation is contraindicated. Graduated elastic compression stockings should also be employed along with leg elevation for DVT. With PTE, analgesia for pleuritic pain and oxygen are often required. Traditionally, UFH has been used in the initial management of VTE[136]. In non-pregnant patients with clinically suspected PTE, treatment with anticoagulants (intravenous heparin and a coumarin) reduces the risk of further thromboembolism compared with no treatment[137]. Descriptive reports show a high risk of recurrent VTE and death when heparin is withheld from patients with suspected or proven VTE, compared with low risks with heparin treatment[138,139]. UFH treatment is monitored by the activated partial thromboplastin time (APTT). Trials of UFH in acute DVT have shown that failure to achieve the lower limit of the target therapeutic range of the APTT ratio (1.5) is associated with up to a 15-fold increase in the risk of recurrent VTE[140]. Use of the APTT to monitor UFH can be technically problematic, particularly in late pregnancy when an apparent heparin resistance occurs due to increased fibrinogen and factor VIII levels, which influence the APTT. Therefore, the use of the non-pregnant therapeutic range for the APTT in pregnancy can lead to unnecessarily high doses of heparin being employed, with subsequent risk of hemorrhagic problems and possibly osteoporosis[141]. In this situation, the anti-Xa level as a measure of heparin dose (target range 0.35–0.7 U/ml) may be useful[138].

The properties of LMWH allow the use of fixed-dose, subcutaneous treatment in the acute treatment of VTE, minimizing or avoiding the need for monitoring. Meta-analyses of randomized controlled trials in non-pregnant subjects have compared LMWH with UFH in the initial treatment of DVT[142,143]. LMWH was found to be more effective than UFH (lower mortality with UFH), and was also associated with a lower risk of hemorrhagic complications. For PTE, LMWH is as effective as UFH in non-pregnant subjects[144]. LMWH has been used for the initial management of VTE in pregnancy[127,145], and has been recommended for this purpose in published clinical guidelines[146].

Occasionally, for life-threatening PTE or where a massive DVT threatens limb viability, thrombolytic therapy with streptokinase or tissue plasminogen activator (t-PA) may be required. Experience is limited, and there is a risk of major hemorrhage if systemic thrombolysis is used around the time of delivery or postpartum.

If UFH is used, it can be given by continuous intravenous infusion or by subcutaneous injection. Intravenous UFH is the traditional method of heparin administration in acute VTE, and may still be preferred in massive PTE because of its rapid effect and the extensive experience in this situation. With intravenous UFH, a bolus of 5000 IU given over about 5 min is employed, followed by continuous intravenous infusion of 1000–2000 IU/h. The dose is adjusted by monitoring the APTT, with a therapeutic target ratio of 1.5–2.5 times the mean laboratory control value[147]. The APTT should be performed 6 h after the loading dose, then on a daily basis. Protocols for heparin dose adjustment according to APTT ratio results are useful as they improve the achievement of therapeutic target ranges[140,148]. Each laboratory should standardize its own target range for the APTT ratio[136,147], and particular consideration must be given to the problems of APTT monitoring in pregnancy[141]. In a meta-analysis of randomized controlled trials, 12-hourly subcutaneous UFH was found to be as effective, and at least as safe, as intravenous UFH in the prevention of recurrent thromboembolism in non-pregnant patients with acute DVT[149]. This route of administration is generally preferred by the patient. When administered subcutaneously, unfractionated heparin is given in subcutaneous injections of 15 000–20 000 IU, 12-hourly, after an initial intravenous bolus of 5000 IU. The dose should be adjusted to maintain the mid-interval APTT between 1.5 and 2.5 times the control value[147].

In non-pregnant patients, once-daily administration is recommended for acute treatment of VTE with LMWH (enoxaparin 1.5 mg/kg body weight once daily; dalteparin 10 000–18 000 U once daily, depending on body weight; tinzaparin 175 U/kg body weight once daily). However, in view of alterations in the pharmacokinetics of dalteparin and enoxaparin during pregnancy[150,151], a twice-daily dosage regimen for these LMWHs in the treatment of VTE in pregnancy (enoxaparin 1 mg/kg twice daily; dalteparin 100 U/kg twice daily up to a maximum of 18 000 U/24 h) has been recommended[145,146] (although there may be circumstances where once-daily dosing, for example with 1.5 mg/kg enoxaparin, may be satisfactory, such as after several months of twice-daily therapeutic LMWH). The twice-daily dose regimens for enoxaparin and dalteparin have also been used to treat VTE outwith pregnancy. One dose regimen for the administration of a LMWH (enoxaparin) in the immediate management of VTE in pregnancy is shown in Table 3.8[145]; the initial dose of enoxaparin (1 mg/kg) is based on the early pregnancy weight, as LMWH does not cross the placenta. Enoxaparin is available in prefilled syringes of 40, 60, 80 and 100 mg. The dose closest to the woman's weight should be employed, and should be continued 12-hourly until objective testing has been performed. Peak anti-Xa activity (3 h post-injection) can be measured by a chromogenic substrate assay to confirm that an appropriate dose has been given. A suitable target therapeutic range is 0.6–1.2 U/ml for peak levels obtained 3–4 h after injection. If the peak anti-Xa level is above the upper limit of the therapeutic target range, the dose of LMWH should be reduced (e.g. for enoxaparin 100 mg twice a day to 80 mg twice a day), and peak anti-Xa activity reassessed. Our experience indicates that satisfactory anti-Xa levels are obtained using this regimen[152], and monitoring of anti-Xa levels can be deferred until the next routine working day, for example, if treatment is commenced at weekends[145]. Indeed, as our experience grows (we have now treated

Table 3.8   The initial dose of enoxaparin for acute treatment of venous thromboembolism

Early pregnancy weight	Initial dose of enoxaparin
< 50 kg	40 mg twice daily
50–69 kg	60 mg twice daily
70–89 kg	80 mg twice daily
≥ 90 kg	100 mg twice daily

more than 40 acute VTEs with enoxaparin), it is clear that this dose regimen rarely requires adjustment, and thus monitoring with anti-Xa levels is probably unnecessary except at extremes of body weight. Great care must be taken in women with a very high body mass index, where it is critical to ensure that an appropriate dose of heparin is used[48].

With both UFH and LMWH, the platelet count should be monitored 4–8 days after treatment commences, then on about a monthly basis to detect heparin-induced thrombocytopenia, which is associated with further thrombotic complications. Pregnant women who develop heparin-induced thrombocytopenia and require ongoing anticoagulant therapy should be managed with the heparinoid[153], danaparoid sodium, or, if postpartum, treated with coumarin with the danaparoid continued until the International Normalized Ratio (INR) is in the therapeutic range. Hirudin could also be used as bridging therapy postpartum.

As coumarins are contraindicated in pregnancy, subcutaneous UFH or LMWH is used for maintenance treatment of VTE in pregnancy[145,154,155]. LMWHs appear to be superior to APTT-monitored UFH in the maintenance treatment of VTE in pregnancy because of their simpler therapeutic regimen. Women can be taught to self-inject and can be managed as out-patients, once the acute event is controlled. Arrangements should be made to allow safe disposal of needles and syringes. Out-patient follow-up for assessment of platelets (and peak anti-Xa levels if required) during treatment should be arranged. Therapeutic doses of LMWH should be employed. In a prospective randomized controlled trial in non-pregnant patients, a 47% recurrence rate of VTE was reported, when thromboprophylactic doses of UFH (5000 IU every 12 h) were employed after initial management with intravenous UFH[155]. The duration of therapeutic anticoagulant treatment in the non-pregnant situation is usually 3–6 months. As pregnancy is associated with prothrombotic changes in the coagulation system and reduced venous flow, it would appear logical to apply this same duration of treatment to VTE in pregnancy. Thus, in pregnancy-associated VTE, therapeutic anticoagulation should usually be continued for at least 6 months. If the VTE occurs early in the pregnancy, then, provided that there are no additional risk factors, the dose of LMWH or UFH could be reduced to prophylactic levels (40 mg enoxaparin once per day or 5000 IU dalteparin once a day, or 10 000 IU of UFH twice daily) after 6 months. Following delivery, treatment should continue for at least 6–12 weeks. Coumarin can be used following delivery. If the woman chooses to commence coumarin postpartum, this can be started on the second or third postnatal day. This will depend on the individual patient, and the regimen for commencing warfarin should be based on local protocols developed with hematologists. The INR should be checked on day 2, and subsequent warfarin doses titrated to maintain the INR between 2.0 and 3.0[156]. Heparin treatment should be continued until the INR is > 2.0 on two successive days.

3.11 LABOR AND CESAREAN SECTION IN THE WOMAN WITH VTE IN PREGNANCY

The woman on therapeutic LMWH should be advised that, once she thinks she is in labor, she should not inject any further heparin until she has been assessed by an obstetrician or midwife. Further doses are usually withheld until delivery is completed. In general terms, where induction of labor is planned, the dose of LMWH should be reduced to its thromboprophylactic dose (e.g. 40 mg enoxaparin once daily) on the day prior to planned delivery. On the day of delivery, the morning dose of enoxaparin should be omitted and the induction of labor performed as soon as possible thereafter. Graduated elastic compression stockings can still be worn to provide some thromboprophylaxis. The treatment dose (twice-daily administration) should be recommenced following delivery.

There has been concern with regard to LMWH and epidural hematoma, through post-marketing reports to the Food and Drug Administration (FDA), largely from the USA. These events have mostly been in elderly women (median age 75 years) undergoing orthopedic surgery. Additional factors such as concomitant non-steroidal anti-inflammatory agent use (which can enhance bleeding risk, particularly in the elderly) or multiple puncture attempts at spinal or epidural have also been implicated. The true incidence of epidural hematoma is impossible to determine owing to lack of denominator data. In addition, practice in North America and Europe may differ, particularly with regard to LMWH use. In Europe, enoxaparin is used in a dose of 20–40 mg daily, compared with 30 mg twice daily in North America. Such differences in patients and practice make it difficult to extrapolate the information in these reports to obstetric practice. A degree of caution must none the less be exercised in the concomitant use of

LMWH and neuraxial anesthesia. In general terms, neuraxial anesthesia is not used until at least 12 h after the previous prophylactic dose of LMWH. When a woman presents whilst on a therapeutic regimen of LMWH, regional techniques should generally not be employed for at least 24 h after the last dose of LMWH. LMWH should not be given for at least 3 h after the epidural catheter has been removed, and the cannula should not be removed within 10–12 h of the most recent injection[157–159].

Individualized management plans are often required with regard to elective Cesarean section in women on anticoagulant treatment for VTE. However, in general terms, the woman should receive a thromboprophylactic dose of LMWH on the day prior to delivery. On the day of delivery, the morning dose of LMWH should be omitted. Graduated elastic compression stockings or mechanical methods can be used to provide intraoperative thromboprophylaxis. A thromboprophylactic dose of LMWH should be given by 3 h postoperatively and after removal of the epidural catheter if epidural anesthesia is used. The treatment dose of LMWH should be recommenced that evening. There is an increased risk of around 2% of wound hematoma following Cesarean section with both UFH and LMWH. Consideration should be given to the use of surgical drains (abdominal and rectus sheath). Skin closure with staples or interrupted sutures allows easier drainage of any hematoma.

A particular problem in obstetrics is the woman at high risk of hemorrhage (e.g. high risk of major antepartum hemorrhage, progressive wound hematoma, suspected intra-abdominal bleeding or postpartum hemorrhage) where heparin treatment is considered necessary because of VTE. She should be managed with intravenous UFH until the high risk of hemorrhage has resolved. Intravenous UFH has a short duration of action, and anticoagulation will reverse shortly after cessation of the infusion should a hemorrhage occur.

3.12 THROMBOPROPHYLAXIS IN PREGNANCY

The management of the woman with a single previous event has been controversial until recently. This is because of the wide variation in risk that has been reported (1–13%)[103,160–163] and concerns about the hazards of long-term UFH therapy, particularly osteoporosis. The higher estimate of risk has led many clinicians to employ pharmacological prophylaxis with heparin or LMWH during pregnancy and the puerperium. However, these estimates of risk have significant limitations. For example, objective testing was not used in all cases, some of the studies were retrospective and the prospective studies had relatively small sample sizes. Brill-Edwards and Ginsberg[164] have recently reported a prospective study of 125 pregnant women with a single previous objectively diagnosed VTE. No heparin was given ante-natally, but anticoagulants, usually coumarin following an initial short course of heparin or LMWH, were given for 4–6 weeks postpartum. The overall rate for recurrent antenatal VTE was 2.4% (95% CI 0.2–6.9%). Interestingly, none of the 44 women (95% CI 0.0–8.0%) who did not have an underlying thrombophilia and whose previous VTE had been associated with a temporary risk factor (pregnancy (35%), oral contraceptive pill (23%), surgery (18%), trauma (14%) immobility (4%), chemotherapy (1%)) developed a VTE, while 5.9% (95% CI 1.2–16%) of the women who were found to have an underly-ing thrombophilia or whose previous VTE had been idiopathic (suggest-ing an underlying thrombophilia) had a recurrent event. Although preg-nancy was a 'temporary' risk factor in this report, as data are limited in this particular area, many clinicians prefer to provide thromboprophy-laxis where the previous VTE has been pregnancy- or 'pill'-related[165].

Thus, in the woman with a previous VTE that was not pregnancy-related, associated with a risk factor that is no longer present and with no additional risk factor or underlying thrombophilia, antenatal LMWH should not be routinely prescribed but this strategy must be discussed with the woman and her views taken into account, especially because of the wide confidence intervals reported by Brill-Edwards and Ginsberg (95% CI 0–8.0%). Graduated elastic compression stockings and/or low-dose aspirin can be employed antenatally in these women. Postpartum she should receive anticoagulant therapy for at least 6 weeks (e.g. 40 mg enoxaparin or 5000 IU dalteparin daily or coumarin (target INR 2–3) with LMWH overlap until the INR is ≥ 2.0), with or without graduated elastic compression stockings (Table 3.9).

In those women with a single previous VTE and an underlying thrombophilia, or where the VTE was idiopathic or pregnancy- or 'pill'-related or where there are additional risk factors such as obesity or nephrotic syndrome, there is a stronger case for pharmacological prophylaxis antenatally. Antenatally, these women should be considered for prophylactic doses of LMWH (e.g.. 40 mg enoxaparin or 5000 IU dalteparin daily), with or without graduated elastic compression stockings. This should be started as soon as possible following the diagnosis of pregnancy. More intense LMWH therapy in the presence of antithrombin deficiency is usually prescribed (e.g. enoxaparin 0.5–1 mg/kg 12-hourly or dalteparin 50–100 IU/kg 12-hourly), although many women with previous VTE and antithrombin deficiency will be on long-term anticoagulant therapy. Postpartum anticoagulant therapy for at least 6 weeks (e.g. 40 mg enoxaparin or 5000 IU dalteparin daily or coumarin (target INR 2–3) with LMWH overlap until the INR is ≥ 2.0), with or without graduated elastic compression stockings, is recommended (Table 3.9).

In the woman with multiple previous VTEs, and no identifiable thrombophilia, and who is not on long-term anticoagulant therapy, there is consensus that she should receive antenatal LMWH thrombo-prophylaxis (e.g. 40 mg enoxaparin or 5000 IU dalteparin daily) and wear graduated elastic compression stockings. This should be started as soon as possible following the diagnosis of pregnancy. Postpartum, she should receive at least 6 weeks' pharmacological prophylaxis, with either LMWH or warfarin. If she is switched to coumarin postpartum, the target INR is 2–3 and LMWH should be continued until the INR is ≥ 2. A longer duration of postpartum prophylaxis may be required for women with additional risk factors.

When prophylactic doses of LMWH are used, the dose may need to be adjusted in women with very low or very high body weight. At low body weight (< 50 kg or body mass index (BMI) less than 20 kg/m^2), lower doses of LMWH may be required (e.g. 20 mg enoxaparin daily or 2500 IU dalteparin daily), while, in obese patients (e.g. BMI > 30 in early pregnancy), higher doses of LMWH may be required. The platelet count should be checked before and 1 week after the introduction of LMWH, then on about a monthly basis to detect heparin-induced thrombocytopenia[165].

The woman with previous episode(s) of VTE receiving long-term anticoagulants (e.g. with underlying thrombophilia) should switch from oral anticoagulants to LMWH by 6 weeks' gestation, and be fitted with graduated elastic compression stockings. These women should be considered at very high risk of antenatal VTE, and should receive anti-coagulant prophylaxis throughout pregnancy. They should be advised, ideally pre-pregnancy, of the need to switch from coumarin to LMWH

Table 3.9 Suggested management strategies for various clinical situations (N.B. special-ist advice for individualized management of patients is advisable in many of these situations)

Clinical situation	Suggested management
Single previous VTE (not pregnancy- or 'pill'-related) associated with a transient risk factor and no additional current risk factors, such as obesity	*antenatal*: surveillance *or* prophylactic doses of LMWH (e.g. 40 mg enoxaparin or 5000 IU dalteparin daily), ± graduated elastic compression stockings discuss decision regarding antenatal LMWH with the woman *postpartum*: anticoagulant therapy for at least 6 weeks (e.g. 40 mg enoxaparin or 5000 IU dalteparin daily or coumarin (target INR 2–3) with LMWH overlap until the INR is ≥ 2.0) ± graduated elastic compression stockings
Single previous idiopathic or pregnancy- or 'pill'-related VTE or single previous VTE with underlying thrombophilia and not on long-term anticoagulant therapy, or single previous VTE and additional current risk factor(s) (e.g. morbid obesity, nephrotic syndrome)	*antenatal*: prophylactic doses of LMWH (e.g. 40 mg enoxaparin or 5000 IU dalteparin daily) ± graduated elastic compression stockings. N.B: there is a strong case for more intense LMWH therapy in antithrombin deficiency (e.g. enoxaparin 0.5–1 mg/kg 12-hourly or dalteparin 50–100 IU/kg 12-hourly). *postpartum*: anticoagulant therapy for at least 6 weeks (e.g. 40 mg enoxaparin or 5000 IU dalteparin daily or coumarin (target INR 2–3) with LMWH overlap until the INR is ≥ 2.0) ± graduated elastic compression stockings.
More than one previous episode of VTE, with no thrombophilia and not on long-term anticoagulant therapy	*antenatal*: prophylactic doses of LMWH (e.g. 40 mg enoxaparin or 5000 IU dalteparin daily) + graduated elastic compression stockings. *postpartum*: anticoagulant therapy for at least 6 weeks (e.g. 40 mg enoxaparin or 5000 IU dalteparin daily or coumarin (target INR 2–3) with LMWH overlap until the INR is ≥ 2.0) + graduated elastic compression stockings.

continued …

Table 3.9 *continued*

Clinical situation	Suggested management
Previous episode(s) of VTE in women receiving long-term anticoagulants (e.g. with underlying thrombophilia)	*antenatal*: switch from oral anticoagulants to LMWH therapy (e.g. enoxaparin 0.5–1 mg/kg 12-hourly or dalteparin 50–100 IU/kg 12-hourly) by 6 weeks' gestation + graduated elastic compression stockings *postpartum*: resume long-term anticoagulants with LMWH overlap until INR in pre-pregnancy therapeutic range + graduated elastic compression stockings
Thrombophilia (confirmed laboratory abnormality) but no prior VTE	*antenatal*: surveillance or prophylactic LMWH ± graduated elastic compression stockings. The indication for pharmacological prophylaxis in the antenatal period is stronger in AT-deficient women than with the other thrombophilias, in symptomatic kindred compared to asymptomatic kindred and also where additional risk factors are present *postpartum*: anticoagulant therapy for at least 6 weeks (e.g. 40 mg enoxaparin or 5000 IU dalteparin daily or coumarin (target INR 2–3) with LMWH overlap until the INR is ≥ 2.0) ± graduated elastic compression stockings
Following Cesarean section or vaginal delivery	carry out risk assessment for VTE if additional risk factors such as emergency section in labor, age over 35 years, high BMI, etc. present then consider LMWH thromboprophylaxis (e.g. 40 mg enoxaparin or 5000 IU dalteparin) ± graduated elastic compression stockings

VTE, venous thromboembolism; LMWH, low-molecular-weight heparin; INR, International Normalized Ratio; AT, antithrombin as soon as pregnancy is confirmed. The dose of heparin given should be closer to that used for the treatment of VTE rather than that used for prophylaxis (e.g. enoxaparin 0.5–1 mg/kg 12-hourly or dalteparin 50–100 IU/kg 12-hourly: note that 12-hourly injections may be preferable to once-daily injections in view of the increased clearance of LMWH in pregnancy), based on the early pregnancy weight[165]. The platelet count should be checked before and 1 week after the introduction of LMWH, then around monthly. Postpartum, she should resume long-term anticoagulants with LMWH overlap until the INR is in the pre-pregnancy therapeutic range, plus graduated elastic compression stockings.

Where a woman has thrombophilia confirmed on laboratory testing but no prior VTE, surveillance *or* prophylactic LMWH, with or without graduated elastic compression stockings, can be used antenatally. The indication for pharmacological prophylaxis in the antenatal period is stronger in antithrombin-deficient women (where LMWH doses of enoxaparin 0.5–1 mg/kg 12-hourly or dalteparin 50–100 IU/kg 12-hourly are usually employed) than with the other thrombophilias, and also in symptomatic kindred compared with asymptomatic kindred. The presence of additional risk factors, for example obesity or immobility, may also merit consideration for antenatal thromboprophylaxis with LMWH. Postpartum, these women should receive anticoagulant therapy for at least 6 weeks (e.g. 40 mg enoxaparin or 5000 IU dalteparin daily or coumarin (target INR 2–3) with LMWH overlap until the INR is ≥ 2.0), with or without graduated elastic compression stockings. These women usually require specialized and individualized advice from clinicians with expertise in the area.

Women undergoing Cesarean section and vaginal delivery should also have a risk assessment for VTE[125]. In a patient undergoing Cesarean section, thromboprophylaxis (e.g. 40 mg enoxaparin or 5000 IU dalteparin) should be prescribed if she has one or more additional risk factors such as emergency section in labor, age over 35 years or high BMI. In patients at high risk, graduated elastic compression stockings should also be used. These can also be employed if heparin is contraindicated. In women undergoing vaginal delivery, a similar strategy can be used, with LMWH being prescribed if there are two or more additional minor risk factors or one major risk factor, such as obesity[48].

Pregnant women now often seek advice on whether they need to take any special precautions to counter the risk of thrombosis when travelling, particularly by air. Outwith pregnancy, long-haul flights are associated with a 2–3-fold increase in risk of DVT, based on case–control studies. The increase in risk is considered to be due to immobility; low cabin pressure, oxygen tension and humidity; and dehydration, which may be enhanced by excessive consumption of caffeine in tea, coffee and soft drinks and alcohol. However, the absolute risk in the non-pregnant appears to be low, with symptomatic venous thrombosis estimated at 1 : 4000–10 000[166–168]. There are no data for the risk of VTE in pregnant women travelling on long-haul flights. However, it appears logical to consider pregnancy as an additional risk factor for VTE when travelling long distances. The Royal College of Obstetricians and Gynaecologists (RCOG) has recently published advice on this area for clinicians[169]. The usual general advice on isometric calf-muscle exercises, walking around the aircraft cabin where possible and avoiding dehydration should apply to pregnant women. Specific thromboprophylactic measures such as the use of graduated elastic compression stockings should also be considered, as results from a pilot study suggest that these stockings can produce a reduction in the incidence of ultrasound-detected DVT when worn on flights of over 17 h duration[170]. The RCOG recommends that, in addition to the general measures noted above, pregnant women should wear graduated elastic compression stockings for long-haul flights. Where additional risk factors are present such as BMI ≥ 30, multiple pregnancy, thrombophilia or strong family history of VTE, medical disorders with increased DVT risk or previous personal history of DVT, pregnant women should wear well-fitting below-knee graduated elastic compression stockings for all flights, and for long-haul flights they may also benefit from LMWH (e.g. enoxaparin 40 mg or dalteparin 5000 U), or low-dose aspirin if unable to take LMWH. However, it is important to stress that women with such additional risk factors often need specific expert advice on the advisability of travel, assessment of their individual level of risk and specific recommendations for prophylaxis. Furthermore, such measures should perhaps not be limited to air travel, as other long-distance travel associated with immobility for long periods of time may also carry an increased risk of VTE.

4

Venous thromboembolism and the oral contraceptive pill

4.1 EPIDEMIOLOGY OF VENOUS THROMBOEMBOLISM AND THE ORAL CONTRACEPTIVE PILL

The combined oral contraceptive pill has long been known to incur an increased risk of venous thrombosis. The first case report occurred in 1961, when a nurse developed a pulmonary embolism after starting the oral contraceptive pill containing 100 µg of mestranol for endometriosis[171]. In the subsequent 40 years, there have been a variety of reports on the association between the combined oral contraceptive pill and venous thrombosis, including case reports or descriptive studies, case–control studies and prospective cohort studies.

Early case–control studies estimated statistically significant odds ratios for the risk of developing venous thromboembolism with oral contraceptive use of between 4 and 8. For example, Inman and Vessey[172] used death certificate information on thrombosis and pulmonary embolism and general practitioner medical records to determine the exposure to the oral contraceptive pill, and compared this with a control group and found an odds ratio of 8.3. A further UK-based case–control study using hospital admission with a diagnosis of deep venous thrombosis or pulmonary embolism found an odds ratio of 6.4[173], while in the United States, Sartwell and colleagues[174] found a statistically significant odds ratio of 4.1 for oral contraceptive users developing venous thromboembolism. There were, however, problems with the case–control studies. For example, they were open to diagnostic suspicion bias, as objective diagnosis of deep venous thrombosis was not widely practiced in the 1960s. Furthermore, the clinical finding that a patient with a suspected venous thrombosis was on the pill could lead to an erroneous diagnosis of venous thromboembolism. It is clear from more recent literature that deep venous thrombosis will only be confirmed in 25–50% of cases at most where it is clinically suspected[105,175]. In addition, it should be noted that these case–control studies focus largely on apparently idiopathic venous thromboembolism rather than secondary thrombosis such as would occur after surgery or trauma. The association with secondary thrombosis was also assessed, and, again, a significant relationship between combined oral contraceptives and venous thromboembolism was found, although the risk was not so great as that found with idiopathic thrombosis[176,177]. A further consideration in these cases was the dose of estrogen used. In the early 1960s, a relatively high dose of estrogen was employed in the oral contraceptive pill, but by the mid-1970s, the dose in the most commonly used contraceptives had dropped to 50 µg, or less, of ethinylestradiol. Further case–control studies suggested a dose-relationship with the amount of estrogen used in the combined pill[178–180].

Prospective studies have also assessed the relationship between the combined oral contraceptive pill and venous thromboembolism. The first large cohort study was the Royal College of General Practitioners' Study first reported in 1974 and subsequently updated[181]. This prospectively studied two cohorts of around 23 000 subjects each, and reported a standardized relative risk of 4.2. Interestingly, despite using such a large cohort, only 30 cases of idiopathic deep venous thrombosis were found in current oral contraceptive users, indicating a low absolute risk. The magnitude of the risk, however, was similar to that obtained in the early case–control studies, and, again, the same limitations applied in terms of diagnostic suspicion bias and lack of objective diagnosis. Other prospective cohort studies, such as the Walnut Creek Study[182], The Oxford Family Planning Study[183] and the Seattle Health Maintenance Organization Study[184] reached similar conclusions with regard to estimates of risk. All these studies in relation to the oral contraceptive pill and risk of venous thromboembolism were considered and reviewed by Koster and associates[185], who concluded that the use of the oral contraceptive pill conferred around a three-fold increase in risk of venous thrombosis. The increase in risk developed immediately on starting the oral contraceptive pill, although it was not related to duration of use. The risk disappeared following discontinuation of the pill.

A more recent study addressing the risk in relation to estrogen dose reported a ten-fold increase in risk, compared with non-users, for women using a pill containing more than 50 µg of ethinylestradiol compared with a four-fold increase in risk in those using pills containing less than 50 µg ethinylestradiol[186,187]. However, there is no evidence that the risk falls further when 30 µg ethinylestradiol preparations are used compared with 50 µg preparations[187].

The issue of diagnostic suspicion and referral bias has recently been addressed. Two studies compared women who were referred for objective venous thromboembolism (VTE) diagnostic testing whose test was positive for venous thrombosis compared with women who were referred for the same test with a negative finding. The relative risk for venous thrombosis associated with oral contraceptive pill use was similar to that found in the population studies, suggesting that the risk of venous thrombosis associated with the combined pill could not be explained by referral bias[188,189].

As well as a reduction in the dose of estrogen in the contraceptive pill, consideration has also been given to the progestogen content. The development of the third-generation progestogens, desogestrel and gestodene, was thought to represent significant improvements over levonorgestrel, as they had a reduced metabolic effect on glucose and lipid metabolism. However, despite these potential metabolic benefits, the third-generation progestogens were associated with an increased risk of venous thrombosis. This relationship was established in three studies published in the mid-1990s[190–193]. The World Health Organization (WHO) Study[190] found that oral contraceptive use was associated with an increased risk of venous thromboembolism in both European populations (odds ratio 4.15, 95% confidence interval (CI) 3.09–5.57) and in developing countries (odds ratio 3.25, 95% CI 2.59–4.08). The increase in risk was apparent within 4 months of starting oral contraceptive pill use. Again, this was unaffected by duration of use, with a loss of the increase in risk by 3 months after stopping the oral contraceptive pill. Interestingly, the relative risk estimates were not affected by age, hypertension or smoking, but, as expected, high body mass index (BMI) was an independent risk factor for VTE, with a BMI of more than 25 kg/m^2 conferring a significant increase in risk. The effect of the progestogen content was specifically examined in a second paper published simultaneously[193]. This study assessed the risk of VTE with low-estrogen (< 35 µg ethinylestradiol) oral contraceptives containing levonorgestrel compared with low-estrogen preparations containing desogestrel or gestodene. The odds ratio for developing VTE in users of pills containing levonorgestrel was 3.5 (95% CI 2.6–4.7) compared with non-users, while the risk for those who were users of pills containing desogestrel and gestodene was 9.1 (95% CI 4.9–17.0) and 9.1 (95% CI 4.9–16.7), respectively. The ratio of the risk of the third-generation progestogen-containing pills to that of the levonorgestrel pills was 2.6 (95% CI 1.4–4.8). This study was also able to adjust for BMI, and, after this adjustment, the estimate of risk compared with non-users was 2.6 for the levonorgestrel-containing preparations, 5.3 for desogestrel preparations and 5.7 for gestodene preparations.

The study by Jick and colleagues[191] examined the relationship of third-generation progestogens to oral contraceptives within the UK

General Practice Research Database. Again, the preparations assessed all contained < 35 μg of estrogen. Consistent with the WHO study, it found that the incidence rates for VTE per 100 000 woman-years at risk were 16.1 for women using the combined pill containing levonorgestrel, and 29.3 and 28.1 for those using the combined pill containing desogestrel and gestodene, respectively. This translated to an adjusted relative risk estimate of 1.9 (95% CI 1.1–3.2) and 1.8 (95% CI 1.0–3.2) for desogestrel- and gestodene-containing pills, respectively. The excess risk for non-fatal VTE associated with these third-generation pills was estimated at 16 : 100 000 woman-years. Spitzer and co-workers[192] performed a case–control study based in Britain and Germany. They reported an odds ratio for VTE for the third-generation pills versus no use of 4.8 (95% CI 3.4–6.7) and 1.5 (95% CI 1.1–2.2) versus second-generation progestogen-containing oral contraceptive pills. However, the absolute risk of death from VTE was 20 cases/million users/annum for third-generation oral contraceptive pill users, compared with 14 cases/million/annum for second-generation pill users and five cases/million/annum for non-users. A further study by Farmer and colleagues reported a relative risk of 1.76 (95% CI 0.91–3.48) and 1.32 (95% CI 0.7–2.69) for users of desogestrel and gestodene, respectively, in a community-based case–control study[194].

Thus, while third-generation progestogen-containing pills carry an excess risk of venous thrombosis, the absolute risk remains modest, and must be set in the context of the background risk of the venous events in young women and also the risk of venous events in women during pregnancy and postpartum, which is substantially higher (Table 4.1).

A recent meta-analysis combining the evidence from all previous studies found that, overall, there was a 1.7-fold increase in risk with the use of the third-generation pills compared with second-generation pills[195].

Interestingly, it has recently been reported that following the so-called 'pill scare', associated with the publicity surrounding the publication of these studies showing an excess risk associated with third-generation pills, use of the third-generation preparations fell from 53% in the period January 1993–October 1995 in the United Kingdom to 14% during November 1995–December 1998. This was not associated with a significant change in the incidence of venous thromboembolic events in these periods after adjustment for age, with the incidence ratio

Table 4.1   Risk of non-fatal venous thromboembolism (VTE) in users and non-users of the oral contraceptive pill. Data from the Faculty of Family Planning and Reproductive Health Care, London, UK, statement from the Clinical and Scientific Committee: Risk of venous thromboembolism and the combined oral contraceptive pill, 15 December 1995

Use of oral contraceptives	Risk of non-fatal venous thromboembolism per 100 000 women/year
Non-users of combined oral contraceptives	5–11
Desogestrel- and gestodene-containing pill users	30
Levonorgestrel- or norethisterone-containing pill users	15
Pregnancy and puerperium	60

being 1.04 (95% CI 0.78–1.39), which would not be consistent with the excess risk previously described[196].

4.2 HERITABLE THROMBOPHILIA AND THE ORAL CONTRACEPTIVE PILL

There is significant interaction between the use of the oral contraceptive pill and heritable thrombophilia. The best studied example is the interaction between factor V Leiden and the oral contraceptive pill[197], showing that the risk for venous thromboembolic events was increased more than 30-fold for women with factor V Leiden who used the combined pill (relative risk 34.7, 95% CI 7.8–154).

This relationship holds true with third-generation pills as reported by Bloemenkamp and colleagues[198], where a 50-fold increased risk of VTE was reported for carriers of factor V Leiden using the third-generation oral contraceptive pill, compared with non-users without the factor V Leiden mutation. Indeed, women who develop venous thrombosis after starting the oral contraceptive pill are considerably more likely to have an underlying heritable thrombophilia, compared with those who develop a venous thrombosis after a longer period of oral contraceptive use[198]. In this study, the risk of women with thrombophilia developing a deep vein thrombosis (DVT) during the first 6 months of combined oral contraceptive pill use compared with prolonged use was increased 19-fold (95% CI 1.9–175.7). The

Table 4.2   Factor V Leiden, exogenous hormones and the risk of venous thrombosis[204]

Factor V Leiden	Oral contraceptives	Relative risk	95% confidence interval
Absent	absent	1	–
Absent	present	3.7	2.2–6.3
Present	absent	6.9	1.8–28.3
Present	present	34.7	7.4–224

thrombophilias included in this study were protein C and protein S deficiency, antithrombin deficiency and heterozygosity for factor V Leiden or prothrombin G20210A. Other groups have confirmed the interaction of risk between heritable thrombophilia and risk of venous thrombosis with combined oral contraceptive pill use. For example, Martinelli and colleagues[199] reported a 16-fold increase in risk compared with non-carriers who were non-users of the combined pill. Clearly, as VTE is a multicausal disease[73], patients with combined defects or who are homozygous for traits such as factor V Leiden are at particular risk[200], as well as those with severe thrombophilic defects such as antithrombin deficiency[201]. Interestingly, although high levels of factor VIII are associated with increased risk of venous thrombosis[202], this confers no greater risk than the sum of each of the effects of the combined oral contraceptive pill and high factor VIII levels alone[203]. To illustrate the interaction between heritable thrombophilia and the combined oral contraceptive pill, Table 4.2 indicates the levels of risk associated with factor V Leiden and the use of oral contraceptives[204].

Clearly, other risk factors for thrombosis such as obesity must be taken into account in considering the risk associated with the oral contraceptive pill. A key factor apart from heritable thrombophilia is clearly a previous venous thromboembolic event. While in the case of hormone replacement therapy (HRT) it is well established that those women with a previous VTE are at significantly increased risk of a further VTE on starting HRT, there are no data for the risk of recurrence in pill users who have had a previous DVT, reflecting that previous VTE has, for a long time, been a contraindication to the use of the combined pill.

4.3 HEMOSTATIC EFFECTS OF THE COMBINED ORAL CONTRACEPTIVE PILL

Clearly, the most likely mechanism explaining this increased risk of VTE is the changes provoked by the oral contraceptive pill on the hemostatic and fibrinolytic systems. There is an increase in levels of procoagulant factors such as factor VII, factor X, factor XII and factor XIII associated with estrogen use, as well as reductions in anticoagulant factors including protein S and antithrombin[42,205]. As well as these procoagulant changes, there is also an increase in fibrinolysis, which is thought to reflect a reduction in levels of plasminogen activator inhibitor type I combined with an increase in plasminogen[42]. However, the net effect, as manifest in laboratory studies that can examine a global test of coagulation activity such as activated protein C resistance or thrombin generation, is consistent with a procoagulant state, which is not countered by the increased fibrinolytic potential[42,206–208].

Given the increased risk of venous thrombosis associated with third-generation pills in epidemiological studies, it is possible that the use of third-generation progestogens alters the effects of the combined pill on the hemostatic and fibrinolytic systems. This has been borne out in laboratory studies. For example, the assessment of endogenous thrombin potential in users of third-generation oral contraceptives shows a prothrombotic abnormality in the coagulation pathways comparable to that found in patients heterozygous for factor V Leiden[209]. In addition to the increase in the endogenous thrombin potential, higher levels of factor VII and greater reductions in protein S have also been reported with third-generation pills compared with second-generation pills[210,211].

4.4 IMPLICATIONS FOR PRACTICE

Clearly, women embarking, or continuing, on oral contraception should be asked about a personal past history of venous thrombosis or a family history of venous thrombosis (Table 4.3). Thrombophilia screening should be available for those patients with a positive personal or family history of thrombosis. It should be noted, however, that there is not a case for universal screening of women for thrombophilia prior to embarking on oral contraceptive pill use. Indeed, it has been calculated that to protect one woman from fatal pulmonary thrombembolism, almost half-a-million women would have to be screened to identify the

Table 4.3   Practical implications for the use of oral contraceptive pills (OCPs) in women at increased risk of venous thromboembolism (VTE)[165]

Women starting the combined OCP should be advised of the small absolute increased risk of VTE. They should have a personal and family history taken of VTE and of additional risk factors for thromboembolic disease (e.g. high BMI)

A personal history of VTE is a contraindication to the use of combined OCPs

A history of VTE in a first-degree family member is a relative contraindication to the use of combined OCPs, irrespective of the results of thrombophilia screening

In current (or recent) combined OCP users undergoing surgery, it is recommended that clinicians:

- Discuss the balance of risks and benefits with the patient when considering stopping the combined OCP prior to elective surgery

- Arrange adequate alternative contraception if the combined OCP is to be discontinued

- Consider specific antithrombotic prophylaxis according to overall risk factors

- Give VTE prophylaxis routinely in emergency surgery

BMI, body mass index; HRT, hormone replacement therapy

20 000–25 000 in European populations who would test positive for factor V Leiden[212]. Clearly, many of these women would be denied use of the oral contraceptive pill, and possibly be exposed to the increased risk of VTE associated with pregnancy. A personal history of venous thromboembolism should be regarded as a contraindication to the use of the combined oral contraceptive pill. A history of VTE in a first-degree family member is also a relative contraindication to use of the combined pill, irrespective of the result of thrombophilia screening. This is because thrombophilia screening will only identify those thrombophilias that are already known and being screened for, and it is clear that there are thrombophilic conditions that may not yet be readily detectable on laboratory testing. Clearly, where the woman is found to have an underlying thrombophilia, she would be best advised to use an alternative form of contraception.

At the first time of prescription of the oral contraceptive pill, it would be usual to provide a preparation of no more than 35 µg ethinylestradiol containing a second-generation progestogen, such as 150 µg of levonorgestrel or 1 mg of norethisterone. This excludes situations such as patients on enzyme-inducing anticonvulsant therapy, where a higher dose of estrogen would be specifically indicated. The risk of VTE should be explained to women starting the pill, but this should be set in the context of the overall safety of the preparation, and the low relative and absolute risk of VTE in patients with no additional risk factors.

For patients taking the oral contraceptive pill who require surgery, there is significant controversy over whether the combined pill should be stopped before major surgery[213]. There are very few data on the risk of VTE following surgery in pill users. The risk of postoperative VTE has been reported not to be significantly different between pill users and non-pill users (approximately 1% vs 0.5%). The small absolute excess risk in combined pill users has to be balanced against the risk of stopping the pill 4–6 weeks prior to surgery, including those risks of unwanted pregnancy, the effects of surgery and anesthesia on such a pregnancy and the risks of a subsequent termination if performed. Clearly, this is a decision that must be discussed with the patient, and if a decision is made to stop the combined oral contraceptive pill prior to surgery, adequate alternative contraceptive measures should be arranged until the pill can be restarted. Although each case should be judged according to the patient's overall risk of venous thrombosis, the use of specific forms of prophylaxis, such as a low-molecular-weight heparin in the postoperative period, should be considered, particularly in emergency surgery or in women with additional risk factors[213].

With regard to progestogen-only contraceptives, which can be used as an alternative in women where the combined pill is contraindicated, it should be noted that there is no evidence that such preparations are associated with an increased risk of thrombosis, or that they should be stopped routinely prior to elective surgery. In contrast, the use of higher doses of progestogens, such as for the management of menstrual dysfunction, is associated with a 5–6-fold increase in risk of VTE[214,215].

5

Venous thromboembolism and hormone replacement therapy

5.1 EPIDEMIOLOGY OF VENOUS THROMBOEMBOLISM AND HORMONE REPLACEMENT THERAPY

Hormone replacement therapy (HRT), in contrast to estrogen-containing oral contraceptive pills which have long been recognized to carry an excess risk of venous thromboembolism (VTE)[192,216], was not[217–222] until recently considered to be associated with such a risk. Although there had been two small descriptive studies that suggested a link, this was not borne out by a case–control study[217]. Thus, clinicians were reassured. However, many of the initial studies assessing the risk had limited statistical power or methodological limitations. Factors such as a lack of objective diagnosis coupled with less reliable diagnostic tools, potential patient selection bias and the less widespread use of HRT are likely to have played a role in the failure to find an association.

Since 1996, a series of case–control studies have shown a modest (2–4-fold) increase in the relative risk of VTE in women using estrogen-containing HRT (Table 5.1). A population-based nested case–control study over the period 1980–94 from the USA reported that women with idiopathic VTE had a relative risk of 3.6 (95% confidence interval (CI) 1.6–7.8) for VTE with current use of HRT, compared with non-users[223]. The absolute risk was estimated at 9 per 100 000 women per year in non-users compared with 32 per 100 000 women per year in users. A hospital-based case–control study[224] set in the UK in 1993–94, assessed 45–64-year-old women with idiopathic VTE. This study reported an odds ratio for current HRT use of 3.5 (95% CI 1.8–7.0) compared with non-users. Furthermore, the risk was highest among short-term current users. The estimate of absolute risk was 11 per 100 000 women per year for non-users and 27 per 100 000 women per year for current users. The well-known Nurses' Health Cohort study from the USA (1976–92) estimated the adjusted relative risk of primary idiopathic pulmonary embolism to be 2.1 (95% CI 1.2–3.8) for current HRT users[225]. A further UK study utilized the General Practice Research Database to conduct a population-based case–control study and found an adjusted odds ratio of VTE for current users of 2.1 (95% CI 1.4–3.2) relative to non-users[226]. In this study, the increase in risk was restricted to the first year of use, with an odds ratio of 4.6 (2.5–8.4) during the first 6 months. Varas-Lorenzo and colleagues[227] reported an Italian case–control study that found a relative risk of idiopathic VTE of

Table 5.1   Case–control studies showing the association between hormone replacement therapy (HRT) and venous thromboembolism (VTE)

Report authors	Study design	Relative risk	Absolute risk
Jick et al.[223]	population-based nested case–control study of idiopathic VTE in the USA 1980–94	2.1–6.9 dependent on dose for current users for idiopathic VTE	9/100 000 vs. 32/100 000 women/year for non-users/users of HRT
Daly et al.[224]	UK hospital-based case–control study in women aged 45–64 with idiopathic VTE in 1993–94	3.5 (95% CI 1.8–7.0) for idiopathic VTE in current users (risk appeared higher in short-term current users)	11/100 000 vs. 27/100 000 women/year for non-users/users of HRT
Grodstein et al.[225]	questionnaire study on primary PTE in Nurses' Health Cohort in USA 1976–92	2.1 (95% CI 1.2–3.8) for idiopathic primary PTE in current users	8/100 000 vs. 14/100 000 women/year for non-users/users of HRT
Gutthann et al.[226]	population-based nested case–control study in UK using the General Practice Research Database	2.1 (95% CI 1.4–3.2) for current users for idio- pathic VTE 4.6 (95% CI 2.5–8.4) during the first 6 months of use	11/100 000 vs. 23/100 000 women/year for non-users/users of HRT
Varas-Lorenzo et al.[227]	case–control study in Italy	2.3 (95% CI 1.0–5.3) for current users for idio- pathic VTE	< 20/100 000 vs. < 60/100 000 women/year for non-users/users of HRT

continued …

2.3 (95% CI 1.0–5.3) for HRT users, with the effect restricted to the first year of use.

The Heart and Estrogen/progestin Replacement Study (HERS), a randomized controlled trial on the secondary prevention of coronary artery disease using HRT (containing conjugated equine estrogens 0.625 mg/day and medroxyprogesterone acetate 2.5 mg/day), studied 2763 postmenopausal women between 44 and 79 years of age who had

Table 5.1 continued

Report authors	Study design	Relative risk	Absolute risk
Grady et al.[228] Hulley et al.[229]	randomized, double-blind placebo-controlled trial of HRT (conjugated equine estrogens and medroxyprogesterone acetate) for secondary prevention of coronary heart disease in USA	VTE: 2.7 (95% CI 1.4–5.0), DVT: 2.8 (95% CI 1.3–6.0), PTE: 2.8 (95% CI 0.9–8.7), for current users (an increase in risk of coronary events in women in the first 4 months of use followed by a reduction in risk over the last 2 years of this trial, which was conducted over 4.1 years, was reported)	230 vs. 620/ 100 000 woman-years for non-users vs. users (reflects older higher-risk population compared with the above studies)
Hoibraaten et al.[230]	population-based case–control study in 1990–96 for VTE in Scandinavia using estradiol-based HRT in women aged 44–70 years	1.22 (95% CI 0.76–1.94) overall, 3.54 (95% CI 1.54–8.2) in first 12 months of use and 0.66 (95% CI 0.39–1.10) after the first year of use for primary and secondary VTE	not available
Writing Group for the Women's Health Initiative Investigators[231]	randomized, placebo controlled trial of oral HRT (conjugated estrogens and medoxyprogesterone acetate in postmenopausal women aged 50–79 years	VTE: 2.11 (95% CI 1.26–3.55) DVT: 2.07 (95% CI 1.14–3.74) PTE: 2.13 (95% CI 0.99–4.56) (an increase in risk of coronary heart disease, stroke and breast cancer was reported)	160 vs 340/100 000 woman-years for non-users vs. users

PTE, pulmonary thromboembolism; CI, confidence interval; DVT, deep vein thrombosis

established coronary artery disease and who had not had a hysterectomy. Women with recent coronary events, recent HRT use, a history of VTE, breast or endometrial cancer, uncontrolled hypertension or diabetes were excluded. This study reported an increase in risk of coronary events in women in the first 4 months of use followed by a reduction in risk over the last 2 years of this trial, which was conducted over 4.1 years. An increase in relative risk of VTE of 2.7 (95% CI 1.4–5.5.1) was found[228,229]. Thus, these data indicate that in older women with coronary artery disease, HRT increases the risk for VTE. In addition, the Women's Health Initiative (WHI) study in the USA (www.nhlbi.nih.gov/whi/hrt.htm), which is a placebo-controlled trial of oral estrogen plus progestogen, or estrogen alone, in younger, generally healthy postmenopausal women, has recently reported its results. This study assessed the major health benefit of oral HRT (0.625 mg conjugated equine estrogens and 2.5 mg medroxyprogesterone acetate daily) in a randomized placebo-controlled clinical trial with more than 8000 women in each arm. The primary outcome measure was coronary heart disease. After 5.2 years of follow-up, the trial was stopped as there was an increased risk of coronary heart disease (hazard ratio 1.29 (95% CI 1.02–1.63)), stroke (hazard ratio 1.41 (95% CI 1.07–1.85)) and breast cancer (hazard ratio 1.26 (95% CI 1.0–1.59)), as well as the expected increase in risk of pulmonary embolism (hazard ratio 2.13 (95% CI 1.39–3.25)). The overall health risks from HRT in this study exceeded the gains from reduced hip fracture and reduced risk of colorectal cancer, indicating that such combined oral HRT should not be prescribed for the primary prevention of arterial disease[231].

Several other randomized trials have also found no benefits of HRT on clinical manifestations of atherosclerosis[232]. However, the situation has been somewhat confused by the recent publication of a cohort study of diabetic women[233], which found that current oral HRT use was associated with a reduced risk (relative hazard 0.84, 95% CI 0.72–0.98) of myocardial infarction. The benefit in terms of protection from myocardial infarction was associated with doses of conjugated estrogen of ≤ 0.625 mg but not with higher doses (> 0.625 mg), and with HRT use for longer than 1 year. For women with a recent myocardial infarction, however, HRT increased the risk of re-infarction. The difference in results between studies on HRT and arterial disease reflects in part the differences that can arise between an observational cohort and a randomized controlled trial[232]. The effects of estrogen replacement on the cardiovascular system may also be more complex than were previously assumed and may vary with dose and timing of therapy in relation to the development of vascular disease.

Hoibraaten and colleagues reported a Norwegian population-based case–control study for VTE in women aged 44–70 years[230]. They found that HRT preparations containing only estradiol had no overall association with VTE, with an adjusted odds ratio of 1.22 (95% CI 0.76–1.94). However, stratification by duration of exposure found that there was a significantly increased risk in the first year (odds ratio 3.54, 95% CI 1.54–8.2) reducing after the first year of use (0.66, 95% CI 0.39–1.10). This study differed from the others in several respects. First, it studied only estradiol-containing HRT and, second, in contrast with previous studies that had excluded cases with presumed risk factors such as surgery, previous VTE and bed-rest, it did not select the women, except for excluding cancer-related VTE. Although this study differed from the others with regard to the overall risk of VTE, it was consistent with regard to an excess risk occurring in the first year of use (Table 5.1).

Thus, the evidence consistently shows a modest increase in relative risk of VTE, although the absolute risk, particularly in the absence of other risk factors, is low. For example, in the study reported by Daly and colleagues, the absolute risk was estimated at 11 per 100 000 women per year in non-users, compared with 27 per 100 000 women per year in users[224]. However, in the HERS trial, although the relative risk was similar to the other case–control studies, the absolute risk was much higher (current users 620/100 000 vs. non-users 230/100 000). This was because the population was at much greater risk of VTE, as many factors and problems associated with coronary artery disease are also risk factors for venous disease, for example age, immobility, obesity and cardiac failure.

There is also a clear association with duration of use (Table 5.2). The highest risk occurs in the first 6–12 months of use. It is interesting to note that the study by Varas-Lorenzo and colleagues[227] reported no cases of VTE after the first 12 months of use.

The dose of estrogen and the route of administration may also influence the risk of VTE. Grodstein and associates[225] reported that the relative risk of VTE increased from 3.3 (95% CI 1.4–7.8) with 0.625 mg, to 6.9 (95% CI 1.5–33.0) with 1.25 mg estrogen. These were consistent with the data reported by Daly and colleagues[224] but this dose relationship was not reported in all studies[223]. Transdermal therapy may carry a lower risk, although data are very limited (Table 5.3). For example, Daly and colleagues[224] reported a relative risk of 4.6 (95% CI 2.1–10.1) with oral therapy, compared with 2.0 (95% CI 0.5–7.6) with transdermal administration. These epidemiological data do not cover all the routes of administration and combinations of estrogen and progestogens used in modern HRT preparations (Table 5.4). Thus, there is a need to extraplolate from the existing data on the effects of exogenous estrogen.

Epidemiological studies have limitations such as diagnostic suspicion bias and patient selection bias. For example, the established association between the pill and arterial and venous thrombosis might influence a practitioner to avoid HRT in women with vascular risk factors. In addition, over the past 10–15 years, our understanding and knowledge of the pathogenesis of VTE have increased, with the identification of a number of new thrombophilic defects that might interact with HRT to enhance the level of risk. Women with such prothrombotic traits are more at risk of VTE, and may have been excluded from HRT prescription because of

Table 5.2   Risk of venous thromboembolism (VTE) with duration of use of hormone replacement therapy (HRT)

Study	Duration of use (months)	Relative risk	95% Confidence interval
Jick et al.[223]	< 12	6.7	1.5–30.8
	12–60	2.8	0.6–11.7
Grodstein et al.[225]	< 60	2.6	1.2–5.2
	> 60	1.9	0.9–4.0
Daly et al.[224]	< 12	6.7	2.1–21.3
	13–24	4.4	1.6–11.9
	25–60	1.9	0.5–7.8
	> 60	2.1	0.8–6.1
Gutthann et al.[226]	< 6	4.6	2.5–8.4
	7–12	3.0	1.4–6.5
	> 12	1.1	0.6–2.1
Hoibraaten et al.[230]	<12	3.5	1.5–8.2
	> 12	0.7	0.4–1.1

Table 5.3   Risk of venous thromboembolism (VTE) with oral and transdermal hormone replacement therapy (HRT)

Study	HRT route	Relative risk	95% Confidence interval
Daly et al.[224]	oral	4.6	2.1–10.1
	transdermal	2.0	0.5–7.6
Gutthann et al.[226]	oral	2.1	1.3–3.6
	transdermal	2.0	0.9–4.6

Table 5.4   Types of oral hormone replacement therapy (HRT) preparations

Estrogen alone: suitable only for hysterectomized women

Estrogen + progestogen regimens: women with a uterus require the addition of progestogen therapy to prevent endometrial hyperplasia

Sequential therapy: daily estrogen is given with 12–14 days of progestogen every month to induce a regular withdrawal bleed. There is an increase in the risk of endometrial cancer with prolonged use of sequential HRT and continuous combined therapy is likely to represent a safer long-term option. Sequential HRT is used in peri- and early postmenopausal women

Long-cycle therapy: daily estrogen is given with 14 days of progestogen every 3 months, resulting in a 3-monthly withdrawal bleed. This is an alternative to sequential therapy with less frequent withdrawal bleeds. The bleeds are often prolonged and heavy

Continuous combined therapy: daily estrogen and progestogen are given with the aim of achieving a no-bleed state

a clinical history of previous VTE. Thus, the case–control studies described above may have been unbalanced with regard to underlying thrombophilia. Furthermore, the index of suspicion of VTE may be higher in women using estrogens than in non-users, leading to more objective testing and diagnosis. However, overall, the consistency of the data suggest that this is a genuine increase in risk of VTE.

5.2 POTENTIAL MECHANISMS UNDERLYING THE ASSOCIATION BETWEEN HRT AND VTE

Effects of HRT on hemostasis and thrombosis

Following the menopause, changes occur in the hemostatic system. These include increases in factor VII, factor VIII and fibrinogen, factors that are established risk factors for vascular disease, and an increase in antithrombin and protein C[234,235]. Oral HRT will provoke changes in the hemostatic and fibrinolytic systems, including reduced plasma levels of fibrinogen, and factor VII, von Willebrand's factor and antithrombin, but fibrinolysis is enhanced through a reduction in plasminogen activator inhibitor type I (PAI-1)[236–241]. However, the changes found are not consistent across all studies, and in particular there is a lack of consistency as to whether these changes in hemostatic and fibrinolytic factors actually lead to thrombin generation. For example, Teede and colleagues[241] reported the hemostatic changes found in 42 healthy post-menopausal women receiving continuous combined HRT with 2 mg estradiol and 1 mg norethisterone or placebo for 6 weeks. This HRT increased prothrombin fragments F1 + 2 and soluble fibrin, reduced PAI-1 and increased fibrinolysis assessed by an increase in D-dimer. However, a recent study evaluated the effects of 3 months of treatment with oral HRT (conjugated equine estrogens 0.625 mg daily and medroxyprogesterone 2.5 mg daily, the preparation used in the HERS trial) and reviewed the literature on HRT with regard to markers of thrombin generation and fibrinolysis[240]. In 12 women who received this HRT for just under 4 months on average, there was no significant effect of HRT on levels of prothrombin fragments F1 + 2, or thrombin–antithrombin complexes or resistance to activated protein C. In the literature review reported, there was a consistent pattern of increased fibrinolytic potential with HRT use associated with PAI-1[240]. These inconsistencies may reflect, at least in part, differences in the HRT preparations used. Interestingly, there is an established association between resistance to activated protein C and venous thrombosis, and HRT is known to provoke an increase in resistance to activated protein C[239,240]. Thus, some of these hemostatic effects appear to be beneficial while others appear to be potentially detrimental in terms of VTE risk.

Inflammation is also a recognized vascular risk factor, and plasma C-reactive protein levels (an inflammatory marker produced by the liver) are increased with estrogen-containing oral HRT[242,243]. Thus, resistance to activated protein C and increased inflammation may be potential mechanisms underlying the association between HRT and VTE.

The route of administration of HRT is also important with regard to effects on hemostasis. Oral preparations undergo first-pass hepatic metabolism, and therefore have a greater effect on hemostatic factors produced by the liver than transdermal preparations, which avoid the first-pass effect. A large cross-sectional study in women aged 40–59 years found that oral HRT, but not transdermal, was associated with increased plasma levels of factor IX, activated protein C resistance and C-reactive protein and with reduced levels of tissue plasminogen activator and PAI-1[243].

5.3 THROMBOPHILIA, HRT AND RISK OF VTE

The risk of VTE increases with advancing age[191,223,224,244] such that the incidence of VTE in postmenopausal women is around double that in premenopausal women. However, in the case–control studies reporting the association between HRT and VTE, the risk of VTE was higher in the first year of HRT exposure. Thus, the interaction of age and HRT cannot be responsible for the increased risk of VTE. This association with the events in the first year of use does raise the possibility of HRT unmasking heritable or acquired thrombophilia. Heritable thrombophilias when considered together have an underlying prevalence of between 15 and 20% in Western European populations, but, as discussed earlier, additional risk factors are usually required for a clinical event to occur.

Lowe and colleagues[245] determined whether a thrombophilic phenotype was associated with the risk of clinical VTE when combined with HRT. They studied 66 cases and 163 controls from the large case–control study of idiopathic VTE associated with HRT, in women aged 45–64 years, previously reported by Daly and colleagues[224]. Twenty hematological variables known to be associated with the risk of VTE were measured. Risk of VTE was significantly associated with HRT use, increased resistance to activated protein C, low antithrombin and high factor IX levels (Table 5.5). Overall, this study found that, regardless of the underlying prothrombotic tendency, HRT resulted in around a three-fold increase in risk. When multiple risk factors are present such as HRT and one or more prothrombotic states, there is substantial increase in risk, with an estimated odds ratio of 153 (95% CI 23.5–1001) for a woman on HRT with increased factor IX, activated protein C resistance and low antithrombin[245]. Rosendaal and colleagues studied the two most common prothrombotic mutations, factor V

Table 5.5 Odds ratios for risk of VTE for hemostatic factors adjusted to include hormone replacement therapy (HRT) status[245]

Prothrombotic factor	Adjusted odds ratio (95% CI)
High factor IX	2.34 (1.26–4.35)
Increased resistance to activated protein C	4.06 (1.62–10.21)
Low antithrombin	3.33 (1.15–9.65)

Table 5.6   Interaction between factor V Leiden and hormone replacement therapy (HRT) with regard to risk of VTE[246]

HRT use	Factor V Leiden	Relative risk of VTE	95% Confidence interval
Absent	absent	1	
Present	absent	3.2	1.7–6.0
Absent	present	3.9	1.3–11.2
Present	present	15.5	3.1–76.7

Leiden and prothrombin 20210A[246], in those women reported by Daly and colleagues[224]. Among the 77 women aged 45–64 years with a first VTE, 51% were using HRT at the time of their VTE, compared with 24% of controls (odds ratio 3.3, 95% CI 1.8–5.8). Among the cases, 23% had a prothrombotic defect compared with 7% of controls (odds ratio 3.8, 95% CI 1.7–8.5). Women with factor V Leiden who used HRT had an odds ratio of 15.5 (95% CI 3.1–77) for VTE. This was a higher estimate of risk than that expected if the risks were simply additive (Table 5.6).

5.4 RISK FACTORS FOR VTE AND HRT

Thus, multiple acquired and/or inherited risk factors are usually necessary for a clinical VTE to occur, and a combination of a genetic susceptibility and physiological, pathological or pharmacological factors such as HRT is likely to be important in the clinical expression of thrombophilias[73]. Therefore, both inherited and acquired risk factors such as age, obesity, varicose veins, previous VTE, deep venous insufficiency, immobility, trauma or surgery, malignancy, cardiac failure, paralysis of lower limbs, infection, inflammatory bowel disease and nephrotic syndrome must be taken into account. HRT should now be added to the list of established risk factors for VTE. This increase in relative risk associated with HRT has to be viewed in the context of that associated with other risk factors. Varas-Lorenzo and colleagues[229] studied the relative risk of various risk factors for VTE, and found that obesity and varicose veins carried a greater risk than HRT (Table 5.7), so putting the relative risk in context. None the less, potentially large interactions

Table 5.7   Association of venous thromboembolism (VTE) and risk factors including hormone replacement therapy (HRT)[227]

Risk factor	Adjusted odds ratio	95% Confidence interval
Varicose veins	6.9	4.3–11.0
Obesity	4.6	2.2–9.7
Osteoarthritis	2.4	1.7–3.3
Age (65–80 vs. 45–64 years)	2.3	1.6–3.2
HRT (current use)	2.3	1.0–5.3
Diabetes	1.9	1.2–2.3
Hypertension	1.6	1.2–2.3

between risk factors can occur. A randomized, double-blind, placebo-controlled trial of HRT (2 mg estradiol plus 1 mg norethisterone) in 140 women with a previous confirmed VTE found that the incidence of VTE was 10.7% in the HRT group and 2.3% in the placebo group within 262 days of starting therapy[247]. The groups were balanced for additional risk factors, including underlying thrombophilia[247].

Selective estrogen receptor modulators

Selective estrogen receptor modulators (SERMs) are non-steroidal antiestrogens. Perhaps the two most commonly used are tamoxifen and raloxifene. There is limited information about the risk of VTE in users of SERMs. Tamoxifen has been used predominantly for its antitumor properties in breast cancer, and there are reports of VTE associated with its use in this situation. The reported risk of VTE with tamoxifen varies considerably from study to study, but overall this is considered to be about a 2–4-fold relative risk of VTE[248,249]. There is also an association with underlying thrombophilia[250]. Raloxifene, with its antiestrogenic effect on breast and endometrium and its estrogenic effects on bone, lipids and coagulation, has been used for osteoporosis prevention in menopausal women. The Multiple Outcomes of Raloxifene Evaluation (MORE) study included 7705 women in a randomized placebo-controlled trial and found that the relative risk of VTE in users of ralox-ifene was 3.1 (95% CI 1.5–6.2), suggesting that the risk is similar to that with estrogen-containing HRT[251]. Thus, SERMs should be considered to carry the same risk of venous thrombosis as estrogen-containing HRT.

5.5 HRT AND VTE: IMPLICATIONS FOR MANAGEMENT

Risk factor assessment and thrombophilia screening

At present there is no evidence to support universal screening for thrombophilia prior to starting or continuing HRT in the woman with no personal history or family history of VTE or thrombophilia. This is because there is limited information on the natural history of thrombophilia in asymptomatic kindred, and the absolute risk of VTE with HRT is usually low. In general terms, it may be useful to discuss the small absolute increase in risk of VTE with the woman (Table 5.8), but it should be set in the context of her particular case. Clearly, in light of recent data, oral HRT cannot be considered to provide the woman with an overall benefit to health, and should usually be used for relief of perimenopausal symptoms. The overall health benefits of transdermal therapy have not yet been established.

Table 5.8   Summary of practice implications for hormone replacement therapy (HRT) with venous thromboembolism (VTE) or thrombophilia[165]

- Women starting HRT or raloxifene should be advised of the small absolute increased risk of VTE, the perceived benefits and possible risks for their individual situation
- A personal and family history of VTE and of additional risk factors for thromboembolic disease such as obesity should be taken
- A personal history of VTE or multiple risk factors for VTE is a contraindication to the use of oral HRT
- A history of VTE in a first-degree family member is a relative contraindication to the use oral HRT or raloxifene, irrespective of the results of thrombophilia screening
- In current (or recent) users of HRT or raloxifene, it is recommended that clinicians:
  - Discuss the balance of risks and benefits with the patient when considering stopping these hormones prior to elective surgery
  - Consider specific antithrombotic prophylaxis according to overall risk factors
  - Give VTE prophylaxis routinely in emergency surgery

It is important to assess for the presence of risk factors for venous thrombosis[213,247,252]. These include age, obesity, varicose veins, deep venous insufficiency, immobility, recent trauma or surgery, malignancy, cardiac failure, paralysis of lower limbs, infection, inflammatory bowel disease and nephrotic syndrome. In particular, a personal history of VTE or a history of VTE in a first- or second-degree relative should be sought. Screening for thrombophilia should be offered if a woman has such a personal or family history of VTE. As in any screening situation, appropriate counselling should be available, including the limitations of thrombophilia screening, and a system must be in place for testing at-risk relatives. It must also be remembered that our knowledge of thrombophilia is limited, and women with a positive family history or idiopathic previous VTE but with no identifiable thrombophilic defect may have an as yet unidentified thrombophilia. In women over 50 years of age with a recent VTE, consideration should be given to the possibility of underlying malignancy or myeloproliferative disorder or connective tissue disease. In the presence of multiple risk factors for VTE, HRT, which is clearly an additional risk factor, should usually be avoided, but the woman's overall situation should be taken into account. In particular, where the woman has had a previous VTE, regardless of whether she has a known thrombophilia, oral HRT should be avoided because of the relatively high risk of recurrence. If HRT is considered necessary for such a patient, transdermal therapy may be best as it has less effect on the hemostatic system than oral HRT. The woman must be made aware of the risk of recurrent VTE. Strategies such as anticoagulant 'cover' can be considered while HRT is required, but the risk of hemorrhage associated with oral anticoagulant therapy must be taken into account. The risk of major hemorrhage while on oral anticoagulant therapy with the International Normalized Ratio in the therapeutic range of 2.0–3.0 has been estimated at 1% per year of treatment, with around 25% of the events leading to a fatality[253]. Women on long-term anticoagulation because of a thrombotic problem need not avoid HRT, and, again, transdermal therapy may be best. These situations merit specialist advice from clinicians with expertise in the management of thrombophilia.

Women with a thrombophilia identified through screening because of a family history of VTE require individual assessment. HRT should be avoided in high-risk situations such as antithrombin deficiency, and with combinations of heritable or acquired thrombophilic defects, for example factor V Leiden homozygotes or women with factor V Leiden combined with prothrombin 20210A or protein C deficiency or where multiple risk factors are present. For asymptomatic carriers of thrombophilia such as factor V Leiden heterozygotes or prothrombin 20210A heterozygotes with no other risk factors for VTE, HRT could be considered, but it is important to recognize that these women will have a several-fold increase in relative risk of VTE. These women can present difficult management problems and should, therefore, be referred to a clinician with special expertise in thrombophilia.

Some clinicians have considered HRT to be a risk factor for postoperative VTE. The only data to support this come from the HERS trial[228]. This reported that the relative risk of VTE was 4.9 (95% CI 2.4–9.8) in the 90 days after surgery for HRT users vs. non-users. This risk was comparable with that for non-surgical hospitalization (5.7, 95% CI 3.0–16.8) and lower than that associated with a lower limb fracture (18.1, 95% CI 5.4–60.4). These women, however, were likely to have multiple risk factors.

In view of the data linking VTE and HRT it seems reasonable to consider HRT a risk factor for postoperative VTE just as we do with other established risk factors such as obesity, varicose veins and immobility, when assessing patients preoperatively. This risk from HRT alone is likely to be modest, and virtually all women on HRT will meet the criteria for perioperative thromboprophylaxis as set out in guideline documents[213,252]. The practice of routinely stopping HRT prior to surgery is not evidence-based, and, provided that appropriate risk assessment and thromboprophylaxis such as low-dose or low-molecular-weight heparin with or without thromboembolic deterrent stockings are used[213,252], HRT may be continued.

References

1. Ruggerri ZM, Dent JA, Saldivar E, *et al.* Contribution of distinct adhesion interactions to platelet aggregation in flowing blood. *Blood* 1999;94:172–8

2. Tracy PB. Role of platelets and leukocytes and coagulation. In Colman RW, Hirsh J, Marder VJ, Clowes AW, George JN, eds. *Haemostasis and Thrombosis. Basic Principles and Clinical Practice.* Philadelphia: Lippincott Williams & Wilkins, 2001:575–96

3. Morrissey JH. Tissue factor and factor VII initiation of coagulation. In Colman RW, Hirsh J, Marder VJ, Clowes AW, George JN, eds. *Haemostasis and Thrombosis. Basic Principles and Clinical Practice.* Philadelphia: Lippincott Williams & Wilkins, 2001:89–102

4. Colman RW, Clowes AW, George JN, *et al.* Overview of coagulation fibrinolysis and their regulation. In Colman RW, Hirsh J, Marder VJ, Clowes AW, George JN, eds. *Haemostasis and Thrombosis. Basic Principles and Clinical Practice.* Philadelphia: Lippincott Williams & Wilkins, 2001:3–16

5. Bachman F. Plasminogen–plasmin enzyme system. In Colman RW, Hirsh J, Marder VJ, Clowes AW, George JN, eds. *Haemostasis and Thrombosis. Basic Principles and Clinical Practice.* Philadelphia: Lippincott Williams & Wilkins, 2001:275–320

6. Stiko A, Hervio L, Loskautoff D. Plasminogen activator inhibitors. In Colman RW, Hirsh J, Marder VJ, Clowes AW, George JN, eds. *Haemostasis and Thrombosis. Basic Principles and Clinical Practice.* Philadelphia: Lippincott Williams & Wilkins, 2001:355–66

7. Robbie LA, Bennett B, Keyt BA, *et al.* Effective lysis of model thrombi by a t-PA mutant (A-473S) that is resistant to α_2-antiplasmin. *Br J Haematol* 2000;111:517–23

8. Stirling Y, Woolf L, North WRS, *et al.* Haemostasis in normal pregnancy. *Thromb Haemost* 1984;52:176–82

9.   Hellgren M, Blomback M. Studies on blood coagulation and fibrinolysis in pregnancy, during delivery and in the puerperium. I Normal condition. *Gynaecol Obstet Invest* 1981;12:141–54

10.   Fay RA, Hughes AO, Farron NT. Platelets in pregnancy: hyperdestruction in pregnancy. *Obstet Gynecol* 1983;61:238–40

11.   Burrows RF, Kelton JG. Incidentally detected thrombocytopenia in healthy mothers and their infants. *N Engl J Med* 1988;319:142–5

12.   Cadroy Y, Grandjean H, Pichon J, *et al.* Evaluation of six markers of haemostatic system in normal pregnancy and pregnancy complicated by hypertension or pre-eclampsia. *Br J Obstet Gynaecol* 1993;100:416–20

13.   Tygart SG, McRoyan DK, Spinnato JA, *et al.* Longitudinal study of platelet indices during normal pregnancy. *Am J Obstet Gynecol* 1986;154:883–7

14.   Singer CRJ, Walker JJ, Cameron A, *et al.* Platelet studies in normal pregnancy and pregnancy induced hypertension. *Clin Lab Haematol* 1986;8:27–32

15.   Gatti L, Tenconi PM, Guarneri D, *et al.* Hemostatic parameters and platelet activation by flow-cytometry in normal pregnancy: a longitudinal study. *Int J Clin Lab Res* 1994;24:217–19

16.   Morrison R, Crawford J, MacPherson M, *et al.* Platelet behaviour in normal pregnancy, pregnancy complicated by essential hypertension and pregnancy-induced hypertension. *Thromb Haemostas* 1985;54:607–11

17.   Burgess-Wilson ME, Morrison R, Heptinstall S. Spontaneous platelet aggregation in heparinised blood during pregnancy. *Thromb Res* 1986;37:385–93

18.   Louden KA, Broughton-Pipkin F, Heptinstall S, *et al.* A longitudinal study of platelet behaviour and thromboxane production in whole blood in normal pregnancy and the puerperium. *Br J Obstet Gynaecol* 1990;97:1108–14

19.   Norris LA, Sheppard BL, Bonnar J. Increased whole blood platelet aggregation in normal pregnancy can be prevented *in vitro* by aspirin and dezmegrel. *Br J Obstet Gynaecol* 1992;99:253–7

20.   Horn EH, Hardy E, Cooper J, *et al.* Platelet reactivity *in vitro* in relation to thromboxane in healthy pregnancy. *Thromb Haemostas* 1996;75:346–51

21. Horn EH, Cooper JA, Hardy E, *et al.* Longitudinal studies of platelet cyclic AMP during healthy pregnancy and pregnancies at risk of pre-eclampsia. *Clin Sci* 1995;89:91–5

22. O'Brien WF, Saba HI, Knuppel RA, *et al.* Alterations in platelet concentration and aggregation in normal pregnancy and pre-eclampsia. *Am J Obstet Gynecol* 1986;155:486–9

23. Douglas JT, Shah M, Lowe GDO, *et al.* Plasma fibrinopeptide A and β-thromboglobulin in pre-eclampsia and pregnancy hypertension. *Thromb Haemost* 1982;47:54–5

24. Clark P, Brennand J, Conkie JA, McCall F, Greer IA, Walker ID. Activated protein C sensitivity, protein C, protein S and coagulation in normal pregnancy. *Thromb Haemost* 1998;79:1166–70

25. Persson BL, Stenberg P, Holmberg L, *et al.* Transamidating enzymes in maternal plasma and placenta in human pregnancies complicated by intrauterine growth retardation. *J Dev Physiol* 1980;2:37–41

26. Halligan A, Bonnar J, Sheppard B, *et al.* Haemostatic, fibrinolytic and endothelial variables in normal pregnancies and pre-eclampsia. *Br J Obstet Gynaecol* 1994;101:488–92

27. Eichinger S, Weltermann A, Philipp K, *et al.* Prospective evaluation of haemostatic system activation and thrombin potential in healthy pregnant women with and without factor V Leiden. *Thromb Haemost* 1999;82:1232–6

28. Holmes VA, Wallace JMW, Gilmore WS, *et al.* Tisssue factor expression on monocyte subpopulations during normal pregnancy. *Thromb Haemost* 2002;87:953–8

29. Comp PC, Thurneau GR, Welsh J, Esmon CT. Functional and immunologic protein S levels are decreased during pregnancy. *Blood* 1986;68:881–5

30. Bonnar J, McNicol GP, Douglas AS, *et al.* Coagulation and fibrinolytic mechanisms during and after normal childbirth. *Br Med J* 1970;2:200–3

31. Booth N, Reith A, Bennett B, *et al.* A plasminogen activator inhibitor (PAI-2) circulates in two molecular forms during pregnancy. *Thromb Haemost* 1988;59:77–9

32. Lecander I, Astedt B. Isolation of a new specific plasminogen activator inhibitor from pregnancy plasma. *Br J Haematol* 1986;62:221–8

33. Nilsson IM, Felding P, Lecander I, *et al.* Different types of plasminogen activator inhibitors in plasma and platelets in pregnant women. *Br J Haematol* 1986;62:215–18

34. Bonnar J, McNicol, GP, Douglas AS, *et al.* Fibrinolytic enzyme system and pregnancy. *Br Med J* 1969;3:387–9

35. Beller FK, Ebert C. The coagulation and fibrinolytic enzyme systems in normal pregnancy and the puerperium. *Eur J Obstet Gynecol Rep Biol* 1982;13:177–81

36. Chabloz P, Reber G, Boehlen F, *et al.* TAFI antigen and D-dimer levels during normal pregnancy and at delivery. *Br J Haematol* 2001;115:150–2

37. Ballegeer V, Mombaerts P, Declerk PJ, *et al.* Fibrinolytic response to venous occlusion and fibrin fragment D-dimer levels in normal and complicated pregnancy. *Thromb Haemost* 1987;58:1030–2

38. Isacson S, Nilsson IM. Defective fibrinolysis in blood and vein walls in recurrent idiopathic venous thrombosis. *Acta Chir Scand* 1972;138:313–15

39. Gerbasi FR, Bottoms SS, Farag A, *et al.* Increased intravascular coagulation associated with pregnancy. *Obstet Gynecol* 1990;75:385–9

40. Kluft C, Lansink M. Effects of oral contraceptives on the haemostasis variables. *Thromb Haemost* 1997;78:315–26

41. Meade TW. Hormone replacement therapy and haemostatic function. *Thromb Haemost* 1997;78:765–9

42. Norris LA, Bonnar J. Haemostatic changes and the oral contraceptive pill. In Greer IA, ed *Thromboembolic Disease in Obstetrics and Gynecology*. London: Bailliere's Clin Obstet Gynaecol 1997;11:545–64

43. Sattar N, Greer IA, Louden J, *et al.* A longitudinal study of lipoprotein subfraction changes in normal pregnancy: threshold effect of plasma triglyceride on appearance of small, dense low density lipoprotein. *J Clin Endocrinol Metab* 1997;82:2483

44. Stiko-Rahm A, Wiman B, Hamsten A, Nilsson A. Secretion of plasminogen activator inhibitor-I from cultured human umbilical vein endothelial cells is induced by very low density lipoprotein. *Arter Scler* 1990;10:1067–71

45. Mitropoulos KA. Lipid thrombosis interface. *Br Med Bull* 1994;50:813–32

46.   Miller GJ. Lipids and coagulation. In Poller L, Ludlum CA. eds. *Recent Advances in Blood Coagulation.* Edinburgh: Churchill Livingstone, 1997;7:125–40

47.   Sattar N, Gaw A, Packard CJ, Greer IA. Potential pathogenic roles of aberrant lipoprotein and fatty acid metabolism in pre-eclampsia. *Br J Obstet Gynaecol* 1996;103:614–20

48.   The National Institute for Clinical Excellence, Scottish Executive Health Department and Department of Health, Social Services and Public Safety: Northern Ireland. *Confidential Enquiries into Maternal Deaths in the United Kingdom 1997–99.* London: The Stationery Office, 2001

49.   Macklon NS, Greer IA. Venous thromboembolic disease in obstetrics and gynaecology: the Scottish experience. *Scot Med J* 1996;41:83–6

50.   Rutherford S, Montoro M, McGhee W, Strong T. Thromboembolic disease associated with pregnancy: an 11 year review. *Am J Obstet Gynecol* 1991;164(Suppl 286)(abstr)

51.   McColl M, Ramsay JE, Tait RC, *et al.* Risk factors for pregnancy associated venous thromboembolism. *Thromb Haemost* 1997;78:1183–8

52.   Kodama H, Fukuda J, Karube H, *et al.* Status of the coagulation and fibrinolytic systems in ovarian hyperstimulation syndrome. *Fertil Steril* 1996;3:417–24

53.   Arya R, Shehata HA, Patel RK, *et al.* Internal jugular vein thrombosis after assisted conception therapy. *Br J Haematol* 2001;115:153–5

54.   Reid W, Perry DJ. Internal jugular vein thrombosis following *in-vitro* fertilization in a woman with protein S deficiency and heterozygosity for the prothrombin 3' UTR mutation, despite anticoagulation with heparin. *Blood Coagul Fibrinol* 2001;12:487–9

55.   McColl M, Ellison J, Greer IA, *et al.* Prevalence of the post-thrombotic syndrome in young women with previous venous thromboembolism. *Br J Haematol* 2000;108:272–4

56.   Bergqvist D, Bergqvist A, Lindhagen A, *et al.* Long-term outcome of patients with venous thromboembolism during pregnancy. In Greer IA, Turpie AGG, Forbes CD, eds. *Haemostasis and Thrombosis in Obstetrics and Gynaecology.* London: Chapman & Hall, 1992:349–59

57.   Greer IA. Haemostasis and thrombosis in pregnancy. In Bloom AL, Forbes CD, Thomas DP, Tuddenham EGD, eds. *Haemostasis and Thrombosis.* Edinburgh: Churchill Livingstone, 1994:987–1015

58. Macklon NS, Greer IA, Bowman AW. An ultrasound study of gestational and postural changes in the deep venous system of the leg in pregnancy. *Br J Obstet Gynaecol* 1997;104:191–7

59. Macklon NS, Greer IA. The deep leg venous system in the puerperium. An ultrasound study. *Br J Obstet Gynaecol* 1997;104:198–200

60. Lindhagen A, Bergqvist A, Bergqvist D, Hallbook T. Late venous function in the leg after deep venous thrombosis occurring in relation to pregnancy. *Br J Obstet Gynaecol* 1986;93:348–52

61. Walker ID. Congenital thrombophilia. In Greer IA, ed. *Baillière's Clinical Obstetrics and Gynaecology – Thromboembolic Disease in Obstetrics and Gynaecology.* London: Bailliere Tindall, 1997:431–45

62. Zoller B, Holm J, Dahlback B. Resistance to activated protein C due to a factor V gene mutation: the most common inherited risk factor of thrombosis. *Trends Cardiovasc Med* 1996;6:45

63. Margaglione M, Bossone A, Coalizz D, *et al.* FV HR2 haplotype as additional inherited risk factor for deep venous thrombosis in individuals with a high risk profile. *Thromb Haemost* 2002;87:32–6

64. Bounameaux H. Factor V Leiden paradox: risk of deep-vein thrombosis but not of pulmonary embolism. *Lancet* 2000;356:182–3

65. Poort SR, Rosendaal FR, Reitsma PH, Bertina RM. A common genetic variation in the 3' untranslated region of the prothrombin gene is associated with elevated plasma prothrombin levels and an increase in venous thrombosis. *Blood* 1996;88:3698

66. McColl MD, Ellison J, Reid F, *et al.* Prothrombin 20210GA, MTHFR C677T mutations in women with venous thromboembolism associated with pregnancy. *Br J Obstet Gynaecol* 2000;107:567–9

67. McColl MD, Walker ID, Greer IA. A mutation in the prothrombin gene contributing to venous thrombosis in pregnancy. *Br J Obstet Gynaecol* 1998;105:923–5

68. Zheng H, Tzeng CC, Butt C, Randell E, Xie Y-G. An extremely low prevalence of factor V Leiden, FIIG20210A and FXIIIV34L in Taiwan Chinese population. *Thromb Haemost* 2002;87:1081–2

69. Den Heijer M, Koster T, Blom HJ, *et al.* Hyperhomocysteinemia as a risk factor for deep vein thrombosis. *N Engl J Med* 1998;334:759–62

70. Greer IA. The challenge of thrombophilia in maternal–fetal medicine. *N Engl J Med* 2000;342:424–5

71. Gerhardt A, Scharf RE, Beckman MW, *et al.* Prothrombin and factor V mutations in women with thrombosis during pregnancy and the puerperium. *N Engl J Med* 2000;342:374–80

72. Greer IA. Thrombosis in pregnancy: maternal and fetal issues. *Lancet* 1999;353:1258–65

73. Rosendaal FR. Venous thrombosis: a multicausal disease. *Lancet* 1999;353:1167–73

74. Conard J, Horellou MH, van Dreden P, *et al.* Thrombosis in pregnancy and congenital deficiencies in AT III, protein C or protein S: study of 78 women. *Thromb Haemost* 1990;63:319–20

75. Pabinger I and the Study Group on Natural Inhibitors. Thrombotic risk in hereditary anti-thrombin III, protein C or protein S deficiency. *Arter Thromb Vasc Biol* 1996;16:742–8

76. De Stefano V, Leone G, Masterangela S, *et al.* Thrombosis during pregnancy and surgery in patients with congenital deficiency of anti-thrombin III, protein C–protein S. *Thromb Haemost* 1994;71:799–800

77. Bokarewa MI, Bremme K, Blomback M. Arg 506-GPn mutation in Factor V and risk of thrombosis during pregnancy. *Br J Haem* 1996;92:473–6

78. Middeldorp S, van der Meer J, Hamulyak K, Buller H. Counselling women with factor V Leiden homozygosity: use absolute instead of relative risks. *Thromb Haemost* 2001;87:360–1

79. Martinelli I, de Stefano V, Taioli E, *et al.* Inherited thrombophilia and first venous thromboembolism during pregnancy and puerperium. *Thromb Haemost* 2002;87:791–5

80. Vincent T, Rai R, Regan L, Cohen H. Increased thrombin generation in women with recurrent miscarriage. *Lancet* 1998;352:116

81. Rai R, Cohen H, Dave M, Regan L. Randomised controlled trial of aspirin and aspirin plus heparin in pregnant women with recurrent miscarriage associated with phospholipid antibodies. *Br Med J* 1997;314:253–7

82. Farquharson RG, Quenby S, Greaves M. Antiphospholipid syndrome in pregnancy: a randomized controlled trial of treatment. *Obstet Gynecol* 2002;100:408–13

83.   Empson M, Lassere M, Craig JC, *et al.* Recurrent pregnancy loss with antiphospholipid antibody: a systematic review of therapeutic trials. *Obstet Gynecol* 2002;99:135–44

84.   Preston FE, Rosendaal FR, Walker ID, *et al.* Increased fetal loss in women with heritable thrombophilia. *Lancet* 1996;348:913–16

85.   Sanson BJ, Friederich PW, Simioni P, *et al.* The risk of abortion and stillbirth in antithrombin, Protein S and Protein S deficient women. *Thromb Haemost* 1996;75:387–8

86.   Brenner B. Inherited thrombophilia and fetal loss. *Curr Opin Hematol* 2000;7:290–5

87.   Dizon-Townson DS, Meline L, Nelson LM, *et al.* Fetal carriers of the factor V Leiden mutation are prone to miscarriage and placental infarction. *Am J Obstet Gynecol* 1997;177:402–5

88.   Meinardi JR, Middeldorp S, de Kam PJ, *et al.* Increased risk for fetal loss in carriers of the factor V Leiden mutation. *Ann Intern Med* 1999;130:736–9

89.   Younis JS, Brenner B, Ohel G, *et al.* Activated protein C resistance and factor V Leiden mutation can be associated with first – as well as second – trimester recurrent pregnancy loss. *Am J Reprod Immunol* 2000;43:31–5

90.   Gris JC, Quere I, Monpeyroux F, *et al.* Case–control study of the frequency of thrombophilic disorders in couples with late fetal loss and no thrombotic antecedent – the Nimes Obstetricians and Haematologists Study 5 (NOHS5). *Thromb Haemost* 1999;81:891–9

91.   Martinelli JR, Taioli E, Cetin I, *et al.* Mutations in coagulation factors in women with unexplained late fetal loss. *N Engl J Med* 2000;343:1015–18

92.   Murphy RP, Donoghue C, Nallen RJ, *et al.* Prospective evaluation of the risk conferred by factor V Leiden and thermolabile methylenetetrahydrofolate reductase polymorphisms in pregnancy. *Arterioscler Thromb Vasc Biol* 2000;20:266–70

93.   Greer IA. Procoagulant microparticles: new insights and opportunities in pregnancy loss? *Thromb Haemost* 2001;85:3–4

94.   Laude I, Rongières-Bertrand C, Boyer-Neumann C, *et al.* Circulating procoagulant microparticles in women with unexplained pregnancy loss: a new insight. *Thromb Haemost* 2001;85:18–21

95.   Kuperminc MJ, Eldor A, Steinman N, *et al*. Increased frequency of genetic thrombophilia in women with complications of pregnancy. *N Engl J Med* 1999;341:9–13

96.   Clark P, Sattar N, Walkder ID, *et al*. The Glasgow Outcome, APCR and Lipid (GOAL) pregnancy study: significance of pregnancy associated activated protein C resistance. *Thromb Haemost* 2001;85:30–5

97.   Alferivic Z, Roberts D, Martlew V. How strong is the association between maternal thrombophilia and adverse pregnancy outcome. *Eur J Obstet Gynecol Reprod Biol* 2002;101:6–14

98.   Morrison ER, Miedzybrodzka ZH, Campbell D, *et al*. Prothrombotic genotypes are not associated with pre-eclampsia and gestational hypertension: results from a large population-based study and systematic review. *Thromb Haemost* 2002;87:779–85

99.   Infante-Rivard C, Rivard GE, Wagner VYH, *et al*. Absence of association of thrombophilic polymorphism with intrauterine growth restriction. *N Engl J Med* 2002;347:19–25

100.   Glueck CJ, Kuperminc MJ, Fontaine RN, *et al*. Genetic hypofibrinolysis in complicated pregnancies. *J Perinat Med* 2001;29:528–34

101.   Clark P, Freeman D, Streja E, Sattar N, Walker ID, Greer IA. The G-to-T point mutation in codon 34 of the factor XIII gene and the risk of pre-eclampsia. *Blood Coagul Fibrinol* 2002;14:1–3

102.   Clark P, Twaddle S, Walker ID, *et al*. Screening for the factor V Leiden mutation in pregnancy is not cost effective. *Lancet* 2002;359:1919–20

103.   Ginsberg J, Greer IA, Hirsh J. Sixth ACCP consensus conference on antithrombotic therapy. Use of antithrombotic agents during pregnancy. *Chest* 2001;119:122S–131S

104.   Hull RD, Hirsh J, Sackett D, *et al*. Diagnostic efficacy of IPG in suspected venous thrombosis: an alternative to venography. *N Engl J Med* 1977;296:1497–500

105.   Lensing AWA, Prandoni P, Brandjes D, *et al*. Detection of DVT by real-time B-mode ultrasonography. *N Engl J Med* 1989;320:342–5

106.   PIOPED Investigators. Value of the ventilation/perfusion scan in acute pulmonary embolism. Results of the Prospective Investigation of Pulmonary Embolism Diagnosis (PIOPED). *J Am Med Assoc* 1990;263:2753–9

93

107. Hull RD, Hirsh J, Carter CJ, *et al.* Diagnostic value of ventilation–perfusion lung scanning in patients with suspected pulmonary embolism. *Chest* 1985;88:819–28

108. Macklon NS. Diagnosis of deep venous thrombosis and pulmonary embolism. In Greer IA, ed. *Baillière's Clinical Obstetrics and Gynaecology – Thromboembolic Disease in Obstetrics and Gynaecology*. London: Baillière Tindall, 1997:463–77

109. Wheeler HB, Hirsh J, Wells P, Anderson FA, Jr. Diagnostic tests for deep vein thrombosis. Clinical usefulness depends on probability of disease. *Arch Intern Med* 1994;154:1921–8

110. Wells PS, Anderson DR, Bormanis J, *et al.* Value of assessment of pretest probability of deep-vein thrombosis in clinical management. *Lancet* 1997;350:1795–8

111. Thomson AJ, Greer IA. Non-haemorrhagic obstetric shock. In Thompson W, TambyRaja RL, eds. *Baillière's Clinical Obstetrics and Gynaecology – Emergencies in Obstetrics and Gynaecology*. 2000;14:19–41

112. Ginsberg JS, Hirsh J, Rainbow AJ, *et al.* Risks to the fetus of radiological procedures used in the diagnosis of maternal/venous thromboembolic disease. *Thromb Haemost* 1989;61:189–96

113. Bates SM, Ginsberg JS. Anticoagulants in pregnancy: fetal defects. In Greer IA, ed. *Baillière's Clinical Obstetrics and Gynaecology – Thromboembolic Disease in Obstetrics and Gynaecology*. London: Baillière Tindall, 1997:479–88

114. Vitale N, De Feo M, De Santo LS, *et al.* Dose-dependent fetal complications of warfarin in pregnant women with mechanical heart valves. *J Am Coll Cardiol* 1999;33:1642–5

115. Letsky E. Peripartum prophylaxis of thromboembolism. In Greer IA, ed. *Baillière's Clinical Obstetrics and Gynaecology – Thromboembolic Disease in Obstetrics and Gynaecology*. London: Baillière Tindall, 1997:523–43

116. Wesseling J, van Driel D, Heymans HAS, *et al.* Coumarins during pregnancy: long term effects on growth and development in school age children. *Thromb Haemost* 2001;85:609–13

117. Flessa HC, Klapstrom AB, Glueck MJ, *et al.* Placental transport of heparin. *Am J Obstet Gynecol* 1965;93:570–3

118. Forestier F, Daffos F, Capella-Pavlovsky M. Low molecular weight heparin (PK 10169) does not cross the placenta during the second trimester of pregnancy: study by direct fetal blood sampling under ultrasound. *Thromb Res* 1984;34:557–60

119. Forestier F, Daffos F, Rainaut M, *et al*. Low molecular weight heparin (CY 216) does not cross the placenta during the third trimester of pregnancy. *Thromb Haemost* 1987;57:234

120. Sanson BJ, Lensing AWA, Prins MH, *et al*. Safety of low-molecular-weight heparin in pregnancy: a systematic review. *Thromb Haemost* 1999;81:668–72

121. Nelson-Piercy C. Hazards of heparin: allergy, heparin-induced thrombocytopenia and osteoporosis. In Greer IA, ed. *Baillière's Clinical Obstetrics and Gynaecology – Thromboembolic Disease in Obstetrics and Gynaecology*. London: Baillière Tindall, 1997:489–509

122. Pettila V, Leinonen P, Markkola A, Hiilesmaa V, Kaaja R. Postpartum bone mineral density in women treated for thromboprophylaxis with unfractionated heparin or LMW heparin. *Thromb Haemost* 2002;87: 182–6

123. Warkentin TE, Levine MN, Hirsh J, *et al*. Heparin induced thrombocytopenia in patients treated with low molecular weight heparin or unfractionated heparin. *N Engl J Med* 1995;332:1330–5

124. Nelson-Piercy C, Letsky EA, de Swiet M. Low-molecular-weight heparin for obstetric thromboprophylaxis: experience of sixty-nine pregnancies in sixty-one women at high risk. *Am J Obstet Gynecol* 1997;176:1062–8

125. Greer IA. Epidemiology, risk factors and prophylaxis of venous thromboembolism in obstetrics and gynaecology. In Greer IA, ed. *Baillière's Clinical Obstetrics and Gynaecology – Thromboembolic Disease in Obstetrics and Gynaecology*. London: Baillière Tindall, 1997:403–30

126. Ellison J, Walker ID, Greer IA. Antifactor Xa profiles in pregnant women receiving antenatal thromboprophylaxis with enoxaparin for prevention and treatment of thromboembolism in pregnancy. *Br J Obstet Gynaecol* 2000;107:1116–21

127. Lepercq J, Conard J, Borel-Derlon A, *et al*. Venous thromboembolism during pregnancy: a retrospective study of enoxaparin safety in 624 pregnancies. *Br J Obstet Gynaecol* 2001;108:1134–40

128.   Hunt BJ, Doughty HA, Majumdar G, *et al.* Thromboprophylaxis with low molecular weight heparin (Fragmin) in high risk pregnancies. *Thromb Haemost* 1997;77:39–43

129.   Blomback M, Bremme K, Hellgren M, *et al.* Thromboprophylaxis with low molecular mass heparin, 'Fragmin' (dalteparin), during pregnancy – longitudinal safety study. *Blood Coagul Fibrinol* 1998;9:1–9

130.   Lindoff-Last E, Willeke A,Thalhammer C, *et al.* Hirudin treatment in a breastfeeding woman. *Lancet* 2000;355:467–8

131.   Barbier P, Jongville AP, Autre TE, Coureau C. Fetal risks with dextran during delivery. *Drug Safety* 1992;7:71–3

132.   Macklon NS, Greer IA. Technical note: compression stockings and posture – a comparative study of their effects on the proximal deep veins in the leg at rest. *Br J Radiol* 1995;68:515–18

133.   Clagett GP, Anderson FA, Geerts W, *et al.* Prevention of venous thromboembolism. *Chest* 1998;114:521S–60S

134.   CLASP Collaborative Group. CLASP: a randomised trial of low dose aspirin for the prevention and treatment of pre-eclampsia among 9364 pregnant women. *Lancet* 1994;343:619–29

135.   Imperiale TF, Petrulis AS. A meta-analysis of low-dose aspirin for prevention of pregnancy-induced hypertensive disease. *J Am Med Assoc* 1991;266:260–4

136.   Hirsh J. Heparin. *N Engl J Med* 1991;324:1565–74

137.   Barritt DV, Jordan SC. Anticoagulant drugs in the treatment of pulmonary embolism: a controlled trial. *Lancet* 1960;1:1309–12

138.   Kanis JA. Heparin in the treatment of pulmonary thromboembolism. *Thromb Diath Haemorrh* 1974;32:519–27

139.   Carson JL, Kelley MA, Duff A, *et al.* The clinical course of pulmonary embolism. *N Engl J Med* 1992;326:1240–5

140.   Hyers TM, Hull RD, Weg JG. Antithrombotic therapy for venous thromboembolic disease. *Chest* 1995:108:335s–1s

141.   Chunilal SD, Young E, Johnston MA, *et al.* The APTT response of pregnant plasma to unfractionated heparin. *Thromb Haemost* 2002;87:92–7

142.   Dolovich L, Ginsberg JS. Low molecular weight heparin in the treatment of venous thromboembolism: an updated meta-analysis. *Vessels* 1997;3:4–11

143. Gould MK, Dembitzer AD, Doyle RL, *et al.* Low molecular weight heparins compared with unfractionated heparin for treatment of acute deep venous thrombosis. A meta-analysis of randomized, controlled trials. *Ann Intern Med* 1999;130:800–9

144. Simmoneau G, Sors H, Charbonnier B, *et al.* A comparison of low-molecular weight heparin with unfractionated heparin for acute pulmonary embolism. *N Engl J Med* 1997;337:663–9

145. Thomson AJ, Walker ID, Greer IA. Low molecular weight heparin for the immediate management of thromboembolic disease in pregnancy. *Lancet* 1998;352:1904

146. Thomson AJ, Greer IA. *Thromboembolic Disease in Pregnancy and the Puerperium: Acute Management.* Royal College of Obstetricians and Gynecologists Guideline. London: RCOG, 2001 (http:www.rcog.org.uk/guidelines.asp?PageID=106&GuidelineID=20)

147. Lowe GDO. Treatment of venous thromboembolism. In Greer IA, ed. *Baillière's Clinical Obstetrics and Gynaecology – Thromboembolic Disease in Obstetrics and Gynaecology.* London: Baillière Tindall, 1997:511–21

148. Hirsh J, Raschke R, Warkentin TE, *et al.* Heparin: mechanism of action, pharmacokinetics, dosing considerations, monitoring, efficacy, and safety. *Chest* 1995;108:258s–75s

149. Hommes DW, Bura A, Mazzolai L, *et al.* Subcutaneous heparin compared with continuous intravenous heparin administration in the initial treatment of deep venous thrombosis. A meta-analysis. *Ann Intern Med* 1992;116:279–84

150. Blomback M, Bremme K, Hellgren M, Lindberg H. A pharmacokinetic study of dalteparin (Fragmin) during late pregnancy. *Blood Coag Fibrinol* 1998;9:343–50

151. Casele HL, Laifer SA, Woelkers DA, Venkataramanan R. Changes in the pharmacokinetics of the low molecular weight heparin enoxaparin sodium during pregnancy. *Am J Obstet Gynecol* 1999;181:1113–17

152. Rodie VA, Thomson AJ, Stewart FM, *et al.* Low molecular weight heparin for the treatment of venous thromboembolism in pregnancy – a case series. *Br J Obstet Gynaecol* 2002;109:1020–4

153. Magnani HN. Heparin-induced thrombocytopenia (HIT): an overview of 230 patients treated with Orgaran (Org 10172). *Thromb Haemost* 1993;70:554–61

154.   Monreal M. Long-term treatment of venous thromboembolism: the place of low molecular weight heparin. *Vessels* 1997;3:18–21

155.   Hull RD, Delmore T, Carter C, *et al.* Adjusted subcutaneous heparin versus warfarin sodium in the long-term treatment of venous thrombosis. *N Engl J Med* 1982;306:1676–81

156.   British Society for Haematology. Guidelines on oral anticoagulation: third edition. *Br J Haematol* 1998;101:374–87

157.   Checketts MR, Wildsmith JAW. Central nerve block and thromboprophylaxis – is there a problem? *Br J Anaesth* 1999;82:164–7

158.   Horlocker TT, Wedel DJ. Spinal and epidural blockade and perioperative low molecular weight heparin: smooth sailing on the Titanic. *Anesth Analg* 1998;86:1153–6

159.   http://www.asra.com/items_of_interest/consensus_statements/ [Current website with consensus statement on anticoagulants and neuraxial anaesthesia from the American Society of Regional Anesthesia]

160.   Howell R, Fidler J, Letsky E, *et al.* The risk of antenatal subcutaneous heparin prophylaxis: a controlled trial. *Br J Obstet Gynaecol* 1983;90:1124–8

161.   Badaracco MA, Vessey M. Recurrent venous thromboembolic disease and use of oral contraceptives. *Br Med J* 1974;1:215–17

162.   Tengborn L. Recurrent thromboembolism in pregnancy and puerperium: is there a need for thromboprophylaxis? *Am J Obstet Gynecol* 1989;160:90–4

163.   De Swiet M, Floyd E, Letsky E. Low risk of recurrent thromboembolism in pregnancy [Letter] . *Br J Hosp Med* 1987;38:264

164.   Brill-Edwards P, Ginsberg JS for the Recurrence Of Clot In This Pregnancy (ROCIT) Study Group. Safety of withholding antepartum heparin in women with a previous episode of venous thromboembolism. *N Engl J Med* 2000;343:1439–44

165.   Scottish Intercollegiate Guidelines Network. *Prophylaxis of venous thromboembolism. A national clinical guideline, Edinburgh 2002.* www.sign.ac.uk

166.   Hirsh J, O'Donnell MJ. Venous thromboembolism after long flights: are airlines to blame? *Lancet* 2001;357:1461–2

167. Ferrari E, Chevallier T, Chapelier A, Baudouy M. Travel as a risk factor for venous thromboembolic disease: a case–control study. *Chest* 1999;115:440–4

168. Kraaijenhagen RA, Haverkamp D, Koopman MM, *et al*. Travel and risk of venous thrombosis. *Lancet* 2000;356:1492–3

169. Royal College of Obstetricians and Gynaecologists. *Advice on preventing deep vein thrombosis for pregnant women travelling by air*. Scientific Advisory Committee Opinion Paper 1. London: RCOG Press, 2001

170. Scurr JH, Machin SJ, Bailey-King S, *et al*. Frequency and prevention of symptomless deep-vein thrombosis in long-haul (≥ four hours) flights: a randomised trial. *Lancet* 2001;357:1485–9

171. Jordan, WN. Pulmonary embolism. *Lancet* 1961,2:146–7

172. Inman WHS, Vessey MP. Investigation of deaths from pulmonary, coronary and cerebral thrombosis and embolism in women of childbearing age. *Br Med J* 1968;2:193–9

173. Vessey MP, Doll R. Investigation in relation between use of oral contraceptives and thromboembolic disease. *Br Med J* 1968;2:199–205

174. Sartwell PE, Masi AT, Arthehes FG, *et al*. Thromboembolism in oral contraceptives: an epidemiological case–control study. *Am J Epidemiol* 1969;90:365–80

175. Huisman MV, Buller HR, ten Cate JW, *et al*. Serial impedance plethysmography for suspected deep venous thrombosis in outpatients. The Amsterdam General Practitioner Study. *N Engl J Med* 1986;314:823–38

176. Vessey MP, Doll R, Fairburn AS, *et al*. Postoperative thromboembolism in the use of oral contraceptives. *Br Med J* 1970;2:123–6

177. Greene GR, Sartwell PE. Oral contraceptive use in patients with thromboembolism following surgery, trauma and infection. *Am J Public Health* 1972;62:680–5

178. Inman WHW, Vessey MP, Westerholm B, *et al*. Thromboembolic disease and the steroidal content in oral contraceptives. A report to the Committee on the Safety of Drugs. *Br Med J* 1970;2:203–9

179. Boston Collaborative Drug Surveillance Programme. Oral contraceptives and venous thromboembolic disease, surgery for confirmed gall bladder disease and breast tumours. *Lancet* 1973;I:1399–404

180. Stolley PO, Tonascia J, Tockman MS, *et al.* Thrombosis with low oestrogen oral contraceptives. *Am J Epidemiol* 1975;102:197–208

181. Royal College of General Practitioners. *Oral Contraceptives and Health.* London: Pitman Medical, 1974

182. Petitti DB, Wingerd J, Pellegrin F, *et al.* Oral contraceptives, smoking and other factors in relation to risk of venous thromboembolic disease. *Am J Epidemiol* 1978;108:480–5

183. Vessey MP, McPherson K, Johnson B. Mortality among women participating in the Oxford Family Planning Association Contraceptive Study. *Lancet* 1977;2:731–3

184. Porter JB, Hunter JR, Danielson DA, *et al.* Oral contraceptives in non fatal vascular disease: recent experience. *Obstet Gynecol* 1982;59:299–302

185. Koster T, Small RA, Rosendaal FR, Helmerhorst FM. Oral contraceptives and venous thromboembolism: a quantitative discussion of the uncertainties. *J Intern Med* 1995:238:31–7

186. Gerstman BB, Piper JN, Tomita DK, *et al.* Oral contraceptive oestrogen dose and the risk of deep venous thromboembolic disease. *Am J Epidemiol* 1991;133:32–7

187. Bloemenkamp DWM, Rosendaal FR, Helmerhorst FM, *et al.* Enhancement by factor V Leiden mutation and risk of deep vein thrombosis associated with oral contraceptives containing a third generation progestogen. *Lancet* 1995;346:1593–6

188. Bloemenkamp KWM, Rosendaal FR, Buller HR, *et al.* Risk of venous thrombosis with use of current low dose oral contraceptives is not explained by diagnostic suspicion and referral bias. *Arch Intern Med* 1999;159:65–70

189. Realini JP, Aencarnacion CE, Chintapalli KN, Rees CR. Oral contraceptives and venous thromboembolism: a case–control study designed to minimise detection bias. *J Am Board Fam Pract* 1997;10:315–21

190. World Health Organization Collaborative Study of cardiovascular disease and steroid hormone contraception. Venous thromboembolic disease and combined oral contraceptives: results of an international multicentre case–control study. *Lancet* 1995;346:1575–81

191. Jick H, Jick SS, Gurewich V, *et al*. Risk of idiopathic cardiovascular death in non fatal venous thromboembolism in women using oral contraceptives with differing progestogen components. *Lancet* 1995;346:1589–93

192. Spitzer WO, Lewis NA, Heinemann LAJ, *et al*. Third generation oral contraceptives and risk of venous thromboembolic disorders. An international case–control study. *Br Med J* 1996;312:83–8

193. World Health Organization Collaborative Study of cardiovascular disease and steroid hormone contraception. Effect of different progestogens in low oestrogen oral contraceptives and venous thromboembolic disease. *Lancet* 1995;346:1582–8

194. Farmer D, Lawrenson RA, Thompson CR, *et al*. Population-based study of the risk of venous thromboembolism associated with various oral contraceptives. *Lancet* 1997;349:83–8

195. Kemmeren JN, Algra A, Grobbee DE. Third generation oral contraceptives and risk of venous thrombosis: meta-analysis. *Br Med J* 2001;323:131–4

196. Farmer RDT, Williams TJ, Simpson EL, Nightingale AL. Effect of 1995 pill scare in rates of thromboembolism in women taking combined oral contraceptives: analysis of General Practice Research Database. *Br Med J* 2000;221:477–8

197. Van den Broucke JP, Koster T, Babriet E, *et al*. Increased risk of venous thrombosis in oral contraceptive users who are carriers of factor V Leiden mutation. *Lancet* 1994;344:1453–7

198. Bloemenkamp KWM, Rosendaal FR, Helmerhorst FM, *et al*. High risk of venous thrombosis during early use of oral contraceptives in women with inherited clotting defects. *Arch Intern Med* 2000;160:49–52

199. Martinelll I, Taioli E, Bucciarelli P, Akhavan S, Mannucci PM. Interaction between the G20210A mutation of the prothrombin gene and oral contraceptive use in deep venous thrombosis. *Arterioscler Thromb Vasc Biol* 1999;19:700–3

200. Rosendaal FR, Koster TE, van den Broecke JP, Reitsma PH. High risk of thrombosis in patients homozygous for factor V Leiden (activated protein C resistance). *Blood* 1995;85:1504–8

201. Simioni P, Sanson BJ, Prandoni P, *et al*. Incidence of venous thromboembolism in families with inherited thrombophilia. *Thromb Haemost* 1999;81:198–202

202. Kraaijenhagen RA, Anker PS, Koopman MM, et al. High plasma concentrations of factor VIIIc is a major risk factor for venous thromboembolism. Thromb Haemost 2000;83:5–9

203. Bloemkamp KWM, Helmerhorst FM, Rosendaal FR, van den Broecke JP. Venous thrombosis, oral contraceptives and high factor VIII levels. Thromb Haemost 1999;82:1024–7

204. Rosendaal FR, Helmerhorst FM, Vandenbroucke JP. Female hormones and thrombosis. Arterioscler Thromb Vasc Biol 2002;22:201–10

205. Meade TW, Haines AP, North WR, et al. Haemostatic, lipid and blood pressure profiles of women and oral contraceptives containing 50 microgram or 30 microgram oestrogen. Lancet 1977;2:948–51

206. Rosing J, Middeldorp S, Curvers J, et al. Low dose oral contraceptives and acquired resistance to activated protein C: a randomised crossover study. Lancet 1999;354:2036–40

207. Meijers JCM, Middeldorp S, Tekelenberg W, et al. Increased fibrinolytic activity during the use of oral contraceptives is counteracted by enhanced factor XI independent down regulation of fibrinolysis: a randomised crossover study of two low dose oral contraceptives. Thromb Haemost 2000;84:9–14

208. Tans G, Curvers J, Middeldorp S, et al. A randomised crossover study on the effects of levonorgestrel and desogestrol-containing oral contraceptives on the anticoagulant pathways. Thromb Haemost 2000;84:15–21

209. Rosing J, Tans G, Nicolaes GA, et al. Oral contraceptives and venous thrombosis: different sensitivities to activated protein C in women using second and third generation oral contraceptives. Br J Haematol 1997;97:233–8

210. Mackie IJ, Piegsa K, Furs SA, et al. Protein S levels are lower in women receiving desogestrel-containing combined oral contraceptives than women receiving levonorgestrel-containing COCs at steady state and crossover. Br J Haematol 2001;113:898–904

211. Middeldorp S, Meijers, JCM, van der Ende AE, et al. The effects on coagulation of levonorgestrel and desogestrel-containing low dose oral contraceptives: a crossover study. Thromb Haemost 2000;84:4–8

212. Price DT, Ridker PM. Factor V Leiden mutation risk of thromboembolic disease: a clinician's perspective. Ann Intern Med 1997;127:895–903

213. Thromboembolic Risk Factors (THRIFT) Consensus Group. Risk of and prophylaxis for venous thromboembolism in hospital patients. *Br Med J* 1992;305:567–74

214. Poulter NR, Chang CL, Farley TMM, Meirik O. Risk of cardiovascular disease is associated with oral progestogen preparations with therapeutic indications. *Lancet* 1999;354:1610

215. Vasilakis C, Jik H, Del Mar Melero-Montes M. Risk of idiopathic venous thromboembolism in users of progestogens alone. *Lancet* 1999;354:1610–11

216. Carter C. The pill and thrombosis: epidemiological considerations. In Greer IA, ed. *Baillière's Clinical Obstetrics and Gynaecology – Thromboembolic Disease in Obstetrics and Gynaecology.* 1997;11:565–86

217. Carter C. Pathogenesis of thrombosis. In Greer IA, Turpie AGG, Forbes CD, eds. *Haemostasis and Thrombosis in Obstetrics and Gynaecology.* London: Chapman & Hall, 1992:229–56

218. Devor M, Barrett-Connor YE, Renvall M, Feigall D, Ramsdell J. Estrogen replacement therapy and the risk of venous thrombosis. *Am J Med* 1992;92:275–84

219. Pettiti DB, Wingerd J, Pellegrin F, Ramcharan S. Risk of vascular disease in women. *J Am Med Assoc* 1979;242:1150–4

220. Nachtigall LE, Nachtigall RH, Nachtigall RD, Beckman EM. Estrogen replacement therapy. II. A prospective study on the relationship to carcinoma and cardiovascular and metabolic problems. *Obstet Gynecol* 1979;54:74–9

221. Boston Collaborative Drug Surveillance program. Surgically confirmed gallbladder disease, venous thromboembolism and breast tumors in relation to postmenopausal estrogen therapy. *N Engl J Med* 1974;290:15–19

222. Young RL, Goepfert AR, Goldzieher HW. Estrogen replacement therapy is not conducive of venous thromboembolism. *Maturitas* 1991;13:189–92

223. Jick H, Derby LE, Myers MW, Vasilakis C, Newton KM. Risk of hospital admission for idiopathic venous thromboembolism among users of postmenopausal oestrogens. *Lancet* 1996;348:981–3

224. Daly E, Vessey MP, Hawkins MM, *et al.* Case–control study of venous thromboembolism risk in users of hormone replacement therapy. *Lancet* 1996;348:977–80

225. Grodstein F, Stampfer MJ, Goldhaber SZ, *et al*. Prospective study of exogenous hormones and risk of pulmonary embolism in women. *Lancet* 1996;348:983–7

226. Gutthann SP, Garcia Rodrigues LA, Castallsague J, Oliart AD. Hormone replacement therapy and risk of venous thromboembolism: population based case control study. *Br Med J* 1997;314:796–800

227. Varas-Lorenzo C, Garcia-Rodriguez LA, Cattaruzzi C, *et al*. Hormone replacement therapy and the risk of hospuitalization for venous thromboembolism: a population based study. *Am J Epidemiol* 1998;147:387–90

228. Grady D, Wenger NK, Herrington D, *et al*. Postmenopauseal hormone therapy increases risk for venous thromboembolic disease. The Heart and Estrogen/progestin Replacement Study. *Ann Intern Med* 2000;132:689–96

229. Hulley S, Grady D, Bush T, *et al*. Randomised trial of estrogen plus progestin for secondary prevention of coronary heart disease in post-menopausal women. *J Am Med Assoc* 1998;280:605–13

230. Hoibraaten E, Abdelnoor M, Sandset PM. Hormone replacement therapy with estradiol and risk of venous thromboembolism. *Thromb Haemost* 1999;82:1218–21

231. The Writing Group for the WHI Investigators. Risks and benefits of estrogen plus progestin in healthy post-menopausal women. Principal results from the Women's Health Initiative randomized controlled trial. *J Am Med Assoc* 2002;288:321–33

232. Herrington DM. Hormone replacement therapy and heart disease. Replacing dogma with data. *Circulation* 2003;107:2–4

233. Ferrara A, Quesenberry C, Karter AJ, *et al*. Current use of unopposed estrogen and estrogen plus progestin and the risk of acute myocardial infarction among women with diabetes. *Circulation* 2003;107:43–8

234. Meade TW, Dyer S, Howarth DJ, Imeson JD, Stirling Y. Antithrombin III and procoagulant activity: sex differences and effects of the menopause. *Br J Haematol* 1994;74:77–81

235. Lowe GDO, Rumley A, Woodward M, *et al*. Epidemiology of coagulation factors, inhibitors and activation markers: the third Glasgow MONICA Survey 1, illustrative reference ranges by age, sex and hormone use. *Br J Haematol* 1997;97:775–84

236. Lindoff C, Peterson F, Lecander I, Martinsson G, Asted TB. Transdermal oestrogen replacement therapy: beneficial effects on haemostatic risk factors for cardiovascular disease. *Maturitas* 1996;24:43–50

237. Lip GYH, Blann AD, Jones AE, Beevers DG. Effects of hormone replacement therapy on hemostatic factors, lipid factors and endothelial function in women undergoing surgical menopause: implications for prevention of atherosclerosis. *Am Heart J* 1997;134:764–71

238. Koh KK, Mincemoyer R, Bui MN, *et al.* Effects of hormone-replacement therapy on fibrinolysis in postmenopausal women. *N Engl J Med* 1997;336:683–90

239. Lowe GDO, Rumley A, Woodward M, *et al.* Activated protein C resistance and the FV:R506Q mutation in a random population sample: associations with cardiovascular risk factors and coagulation variables. *Thromb Haemost* 1999;81:918–24

240. Douketis JD, Gordon M, Johnston M, *et al.* The effects of hormone replacement therapy on thrombin generation, fibrinolysis inhibition, and resistance to activated protein C: prospective cohort and review of the literature. *Thromb Res* 2000;99:25–34

241. Teede HJ, McGrath BP, Smolich JJ, *et al.* Postmenopausal hormone replacement therapy increases coagulation activity and fibrinolysis. *Arterioscler Thromb Vasc Biol* 2000;20:1404–9

242. Ridker P, Hennekens C, Rifai N, *et al.* Hormone replacement therapy and increased plasma concentration of C-reactive protein. *Circulation* 1999;100:713–16

243. Lowe GDO, Upton MN, Rumley A, McConnachie A, O'Reilly D, Watt GCM. Different aspects of oral and transdermal hormone replacement therapies on factor IX, APC resistance, t-PA, PAI and C-reactive protein. A cross-sectional population survey. *Thromb Haemost* 2001;86:550–6

244. The Postmenopausal Estrogen/Progestin Interventions Trial Writing Group. Effects of estrogen/progestin regimens on heart disease risk factors in postmenopausal women. *J Am Med Assoc* 1995;273:199–208

245. Lowe GDO, Woodward M, Vessey M, Rumley A, Gough P, Daly E. Thrombotic variables and risk of idiopathic venous thromboembolism in women aged 45–64 years. *Thromb Haemost* 2000;83:530–5

246.   Rosendaal FR, Vessey M, Rumley A, *et al.*   Hormonal replacement therapy, prothrombotic mutations and the risk of venous thrombosis. *Br J Haematol* 2002;116:851–4

247.   Hoibraaten E, Qvigstad E, Arnesen H, *et al.* Increased risk of recurrent venous thromboembolism during hormone replacement therapy. *Thromb Haemost* 2000;84:961–7

248.   Meier CR, Jick H. Tamoxifen and risk of idiopathic venous thromboembolism. *Br J Clin Pharmacol* 1998;45:602–8

249.   Fisher B, Digham J, Wolmark N, *et al.* Tamoxifen in treatment of intraductal breast cancer: national surgical adjuvant breast and bowel project B-24 randomised controlled trial. *Lancet* 1999;353:1993–2000

250.   Weitz JC, Israel VK, Leibman HA.   Tamoxifen-associated venous thrombosis and activated proten C resistance due to factor V Leiden. *Cancer* 1997;79:2024–7

251.   Ettinger B, Black DM, Mitlak BH, *et al.* Reduction of vertebral fracture risk in post menopausal women with osteoporosis treated with raloxifene: results from a 3 year randomised clinical trial.   Multiple Outcomes of Raloxifene Evaluation (MORE) Investigators. *J Am Med Assoc* 1999;282:637–45

252.   Greer IA, Walker ID. Hormone replacement therapy and venous thromboembolism. *Climacteric* 1999;2:1–8

253.   Palereti G, Leali N, Cocheri S, *et al.* Bleeding complications of oral anticoagulant treatment: an inception cohort, prospective collaborative study (ISCOAT).   Italian Study on Complications of Oral Anticoagulant Therapy. *Lancet* 1996;348:423–8

Index